Handbook of Acupressure

Handbook of Acupressure

Dr. A.K. Saxena
Dr. Preeti Pai

Ocean Books Pvt. Ltd.
ISO 9001:2015 Publishers

Published by
Ocean Books (P) Ltd.
4/19 Asaf Ali Road,
New Delhi-110 002 (INDIA)
e-mail: info@oceanbooks.in

ISBN 978-81-8430-541-8
HANDBOOK OF ACUPRESSURE
by Dr. A.K. Saxena & Dr. Preeti Pai

Edition
2026

Price
₹ 600.00 (Rupees Six Hundred only)

Printed at
R-Tech Offset Printers, Delhi

Dedication

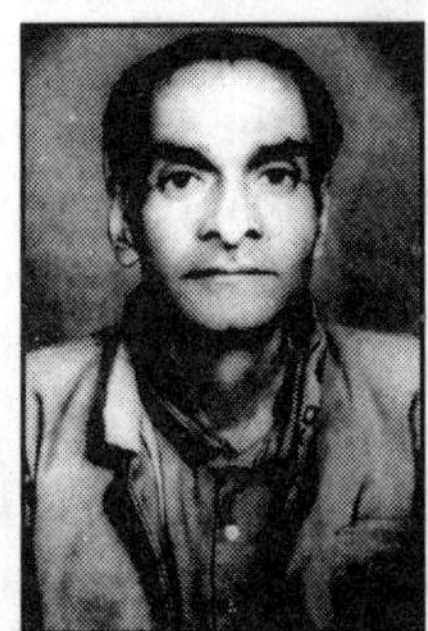

(Late) Shri Vidya Dhar Saxena

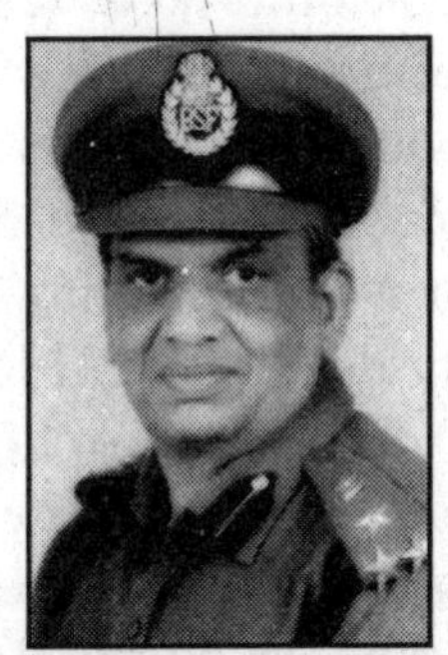

Padamshree (Late) Dr. L.C. Gupta

This book is dedicated to my respected father (Late) Shri Vidya Dhar Saxena, who led a saintly life. He lived for others and always inspired me to live for others and taught me to realise the pleasure in contentment and work selflessly. He left for his heavenly abode on 13th January, 1968, when I was yet to complete 19 years of my age. However, his noble soul has always been with me, inspiring me to do something which could be of some use to the people for times to come.

This book is also dedicated to Padamshree (Late) Dr. L.C. Gupta, former Inspector General of Police & Director (Medical), BSF, my true friend, philosopher and guide. What a great visionary he was and how large a heart he had, can be gauged by the fact that he kindly agreed to hold the hand of an upcoming first-timer author of non-conventional medicine, despite himself being an accomplished doctor of Conventional Medicine, author of as many as Ninty-five books on Medical Science. A person who had begged many national and international awards, agreed to co-author our first book, *Miraculous Effects of Acupressure* with me, which incidentally became one of the best-sellers in the international market. But for his name, no publisher would have ventured to publish my book otherwise. He always encouraged me and authored yet another book with me *Acupressure aur Swasth Jeevan*. He conceived the idea of bringing out yet another book, *101 Q&A Acupressure & Reflexology*, in question and answer form, which unfortunately had to be dedicated to him. My destiny....!!! I lost a great friend and inspirer....!!! Be it writing a book or holding Health Workshops for the benefit to masses, he always stood to support me. In the year 2010, Padamshree Award was conferred upon him for writing 112 books on Medical Science, a world record in itself. He was an institution in himself. Overall, a great human being, with vast knowledge, an open mind, an artist (painting and sculpture) who possessed a great sense of humour and a huge heart full of compassion.

Acupressure Training and Healing Centre

Acupressure is not only curative, it is preventive as well as partially diagnostic too to some extent. This therapy is totally non-conventional, non-interventional, and non-invasive. It is simple to learn and easy to practice. It is free from any side effect as no medicines whatsoever have to be given. It simply works on the premise that human body has tremendous healing power, the role of acupressure is to invoke that healing power in the right direction to attain a state of fitness.

Any one can learn to heal, using this technique. Whereas, knowledge of human body/physiology has added benefit, yet qualification is no constraint in learning Acupressure. All that is essential is the understanding of Hindi or English language in which training is given. Besides, the key factors are dedication to do hard work and a desire to help the suffering mankind from agony and pain. Once you learn to heal using acupressure technique, you can help yourself, your family members, and friends, sitting in the comfort of your home. Even house-wives can learn to heal using this technique. In case you too want to avail this facility, please contact:

Director, Acupressure Training and Healing Centre,
B-702, SHRAMDEEP Apartments,
Sector-62, NOIDA-201301 (Uttar Pradesh), INDIA.
09810484242/09810430343

saxenaashokk@yahoo.com
Website : acupressureguide.org

Highlights:

- Training is given by Dr. A.K. Saxena himself at Delhi/NCR, as also in the sessions organized outside Delhi.
- Training is given by Dr. Preeti Pai at our Pune Centre.
- Three months/Crash* Certificate Courses available.
- Reasonable Fees (₹ 7500/- only, per person for a group not less than eight persons), for Indians.
- Practical training compulsory.

101 Q&A
ACUPRESSURE
&
REFLEXOLOGY

I am amazed go through this Book on acupressure by Dr [illegible] of Saxena. Dr Saxena
I am also taken the treatment with Dr Saxena. I am so happy that he is curing several people in this country and saves the people who are suffering with pain in a [illegible] [illegible]

I wish him well

H D Devegowda
23/12/014

H. D. DEVE GOWDA
Member of Parliament (LS)
No. 5, Safdarjung Lane,
New Delhi-110011
Tel. 011-23794499 Fax: 011-23794431

Former Prime Minister of India

[illegible]

New Delhi
May 11, [illegible]

[illegible]
Judge
[illegible]

Pinaki Chandra Ghose
Judge
Supreme Court of India

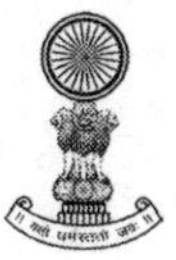

11, Moti Lal Nehru Marg
New Delhi - 110 011
Ph.: 23018043

TO WHOMSOEVER IT MAY CONCERN

Health is not merely the absence of disease but well-being, not only at a physical level but also on mental, social and spiritual levels. The concept of treating the body as an assembly of separate independent parts – hitherto adopted by the medical world – has invisible unit is gaining momentum in all parts of the world.

Shri Ashok Saxena, an Acupressure Consultant has been providing Acupressure therapy treatment as a service to the general public suffering from various ailments.

Drugless therapy offers an opportunity to reduce medicine intake and provides cure for daily ailments. The holistic approach, adopted by such simple therapies, offers the common a wonderful tool to heal himself.

I undertook Acupressure treatment from Shri Ashok Saxena and he treated me for about 10 days with Acupressure therapy and I am very much relieved from my back pain and other ailments. I hope that this therapy should be spread more effectively in our country.

I wish and pray to God to bless Shri Ashok Saxena with long life, thus enabling him to extend his selfless service to all those who suffer various ailments.

Pinaki Chandra Ghose

New Delhi;
May 11, 2016.

(Justice Pinaki Chandra Ghose)
Judge
Supreme Court of India

G. S. Sistani
Judge
HIGH COURT OF DELHI

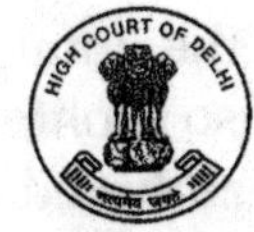

8A, Tuglak Road,
New Delhi - 110011
Ph. : 23793986
Off : 23074203
Fax : 23782731

TO WHOMSOEVER IT MAY CONCERN

Acupressure is a traditional Chinese medical theory. The goal of acupressure or other types of Asian bodywork is to restore health and balance to the body's channels of energy and to regulate opposing forces of negative energy and positive energy. During treatment, physical pressure is applied to acupuncture points by acupressure practitioners by using their fingers, palms, elbows, feet, or special devices to apply pressure to acupoints on the body's meridians. Sometimes, acupressure also involves stretching or acupressure massage, as well as other methods. Acupressure is very helpful in various ailments such as anxiety, migraine, tension, facial pain, neck and shoulder pain, joint pains, lower back pain, stroke rehabilitations, allergies, sinus, congestion, besides various other ailments as explained by Dr. A.K. Saxena.

I met Dr. A.K. Saxena through a common friend, who spoke very highly of him. At that time, I was not very familiar with Acupressure therapy and was always related/ associated it with great discomfort and pain to a patient.

My opinion changed after coming in touch with Dr. Saxena, who treated my mother-in-law for Parkinson disease, and under his guidance she has made noticeable improvement. Dr. Saxena also treated me for my frozen shoulder, which has had amazing results.

I feel that Dr. Saxena is a combination of expertise, God's gift and temperament which leads to exceptional results. He uses his art efficiently giving tremendous results to his patients. I am of the opinion that his art should not only be promoted but also proliferated across India. To this end, Dr. Saxena has co-authored a book called *Handbook of Acupressure* which is an outcome of the practical experience garnered by Dr. Saxena in his years of experience. In this book, Dr. Saxena has incorporated details in the form of case studies with regard to different ailments suffered by various patients and also explained how such patients have been benefitted with the help of acupressure. Dr. Saxena has also explained what should be the trigger points, what is the duration of a session for a particular disease/problem, what should be the dietary regime, besides various *prayanams,* in order to achieve positive and faster relief. I firmly believe and trust that this book would be of immense benefit not only to patients but to its readers.

I wish the Almighty to grant Dr. Saxena a long life to enable people to benefit from his art.

(G.S. Sistani)
Judge
High Court of Delhi

Justice Alok Singh

Bunglow No. 01,
Near Pant Sadan,
Mallital, Nainital.
Ph.No.05942-237151

12.08.17.

My dear Dr. Saxena,

I was told about the expertise of Dr Saxena in acupressure by my wife's sister who was herself treated by him. I have been treated by him for weakness in my right palm and right leg post a brain stroke. Dr Saxena also cured my wife's lower back pain and my younger son's shoulder pain with his Midas touch.

Dr Saxena's acumen and finesse is par excellence and I could see in him zeal to disseminate knowledge about this method of drug less healing of body and mind. Also, his technique to engage the patient in a dialogue while giving treatment reduces the bodily uneasiness.

I have also had the opportunity to read some parts of his book titled "Handbook of Acupressure" which he has co authored with Dr Preeti Pai, who is herself a seasoned and gifted acupuncturist, which made me realize that acupressure is a scientific and holistic way to cure most of the bodily ailments without any drug or intervention.

I wish that Dr Saxena keeps up all his good work and author more books which will benefit a lot of suffering people. May god bless him with great health. My best wishes to him for all his future endeavors.

Alok Singh

Judge, High Court of Uttarakhand

PRABHAT KUMAR
FORMER CABINET SECRETARY
FIRST GOVERNOR OF JHARKHAND

F1, Sector 39
Noida– 201303

The beauty of acupressure therapy is that it does not involve the prescription of drugs, nor does it have any side effects. Besides, it is non-invasive, non-interventional and non-conventional.

The present book is a compilation of actual case studies of the treatment of some of the most intractable and terminal medical problems by the authors through acupressure. While dealing with these difficult cases, even the authors were not too sure about the final outcome. The purpose of chronicling these studies is to share the authors' knowledge with other practicing therapists and students of acupressure. What is most satisfying is to note that the authors have emphasized the importance of co-management instead of advocating the superiority of one therapy over others.

I have been observing the senior author of the book Dr. A.K. Saxena for quite some time as an acupressure expert and have been witness to his remarkable successes in several complicated cases. He has a rich experience in healing various types of ailments for nearly three decades and has been associated with a number of reputed hospitals as a visiting consultant. His co-author Dr. Preeti Pai is also a gifted therapist and has been conducting research projects in acupressure. Together they have co-authored a number of books on the subject.

Needless to say, this volume would make a valuable contribution to the science of acupressure and will be appreciated by everyone.

I extend my best wishes for the success of the book.

(Prabhat Kumar)

Justice C.M. Nayar (Retd.)
Former Chirman MRTP Commission

C – 490, Defence Colony,
New Delhi – 110 024 INDIA
Phone : 011-24338055, 24333132
Email : cmnayar2009@gmail.com

Ref. No. Dated : 27/05/2016

TO WHOMSOEVER IT MAY CONCERN

We have been introduced to Dr. A.K. Saxena by our friend Mr. B.K. Tamini, I.A.S. (Retd.), while attending a common dinner, I suffer from medical problem due to *market central,* lateral canal and foraminal stenosis at L4-5 level with the trefoil shaped of the canal, etc. as diagnosed by MRI of the lumber spine and the doctor attending on the same, and I was recommended surgery. Dr. A.K. Saxena attended on the problem and used the technique called 'Acupressure' and I have already undergone eight sittings. He has very fairly stated that the problem will not be hundred percent cured but major relief will be expected in due course say about three months. Similarly, my wife, Mrs. Asha Nayar, I.A.S. (Retd.) has been suffering knee pain and discomfort and surgery has been recommended as an option. Dr. Saxena has attended on her by same technique and she is feeling much better in a couple of sittings.

Dr. Saxena very ably attends on his patients and engages them in useful and meaningful conversation to enable them to recover physically and provide mental comfort to tackle the problems. I understand he has brought relief to large number of persons by his able hands and kind words. He has perfected the art of Acupressure bringing relief to so many people. This line of treatment is a major innovation as an alternative to even surgery and is required to be encouraged and promoted for the benefit of all. We understand Dr. Saxena is often invited to preside and give lectures in institutions of repute for the benefit of general public.

We wish Dr. Saxena the best in life and pray that he continues to progress in his meaningful pursuit to bring relief to all irrespective of the age group and relieve the suffering of the people.

(C.M. Nayar)

ANOOP GEORGE CHAUDHARI
Senior Advocate
Former Advocate General, M.P.

Dated : 17/04/2017

There are two facets to Dr. Saxena, one as a humanist and second as an acupressurist. In both these facets, Dr. Saxena is non-pareil.

I was referred to Dr. A.K. Saxena by another Ashok, the late Ashok Shrivastava, Senior Advocate, a dear friend. I was told that Dr. Saxena has magic in his hands. I did not realize at that time that I would soon be experiencing that magic. I was treated for a painful shoulder injury and was the recipient of immediate and long-lasting relief.

Dr. Saxena has in the past written books (translated in several languages) which apart from being informative are also immensely helpful in using the technique of acupressure as a means for relieving pain and discomfort.

It is said that health is in your hands and I am sure that this upcoming book of Dr. Saxena will help to alleviate painful conditions and sufferings.

I wish a successful launch of his book.

(Anoop George Chaudhari)

BRIJ K. [illegible] Tel. No. [illegible]
I.A.S. (Retd.)
Member
National Commission [illegible]

TO WHOMSOEVER IT MAY CONCERN

I have known [illegible] years. The relationship [illegible] in late 1997 [illegible] hands and [illegible] advised [illegible] Several [illegible] brought [illegible] listening [illegible] treatment [illegible] called [illegible] day of [illegible] admire [illegible] times [illegible] recurred [illegible]

I have [illegible] professionally since [illegible] student of the art [illegible] and teach [illegible] "Art" [illegible] cases leaving with [illegible] and engaging the patient [illegible] conversation [illegible] real treat. He has [illegible] persons who [illegible]

That he [illegible] pressure bringing relief [illegible]

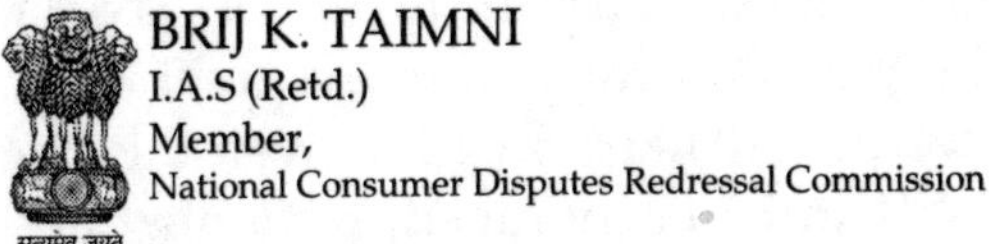

BRIJ K. TAIMNI
I.A.S (Retd.)
Member,
National Consumer Disputes Redressal Commission

Tel. No. 3712458
JANPATH BHAVAN
5th FLOOR 'A' WING
JANPATH
NEW DELHI - 110 001

TO WHOMSOEVER IT MAY CONCERN

I have known Dr. A.K. Saxena by now for over four years. The relationship started in interesting circumstances in late 1997, I started having pain in my shoulder, elbow, hands and fingertips. As the things went serious, I was advised to consult an orthopedic surgeon, which I did. Several rounds of consultation and physiotherapy sittings brought hardly any relief. Then a common friend after listening to my story referred me to Dr. Saxena. I started treatment under his able hand—literally—using technique called 'acu-pressure', as a doubting-tom but by fifth or sixth day of 'sitting' — as Dr. Saxena call it — I had become his admirer and his un-official spokesperson. Those ten or so sitting's has done a 'magic' and that type of pain has not recurred since.

I have come to know Dr. Saxena both- personally and professionally since then. I have found him to be a devoted student of the art of "fingers and toes" ever willing to learn and teach, so that the patient could practice and apply this "Art" at home. I have heard and seen several otherwise lost cases leaving with cheerful gratitude. Seeing him working and engaging the patient in a positive conversation is a real treat. He has brought succor and relief to thousands of persons who are beholden to him like me.

That he has been able to almost perfect this art Acu-pressure bringing relief to them while continuing to perform

Res. : C-II/41, Moti Bagh, New Delhi Tel No. 4102445, 4109851 his other bread-earning duties is a tribute to this Dr. Saxena. That he is devoting his personal time for such a great work. How we wish there were more like him. Moreover, this line of treatment also needs to be encouraged, promoted and popularized for the benefit of all along with other systems of treatment and cure – both traditional/non traditional and indigenous/non-indigenous.

I wish Dr. Saxena all the very best in his life. I am sure that the good wishes and prayers of all whom he treated and brought relief, will strengthen his resolve to still improve upon this. God given gift by picking up new 'modes' from where this art originated and is practiced more widely than is the case of this country.

(Brij K. Taimni)

AJIT S. BHASME

Advocate Supreme Court

Chamber:
336 New Supreme Court
Lawyers Chambers
Bhagwan Das Road
(Opp Supreme Court)
New Delhi - 110001
Phone : 23384019
Telefax : 011-23384019 (On Call)

Mumbai Office & Residence :
By appointment only
14B Samata
Gen. J. Bhosale Marg
Nariman Point
Mumbai : 400 021
Phone : 22873369
Mobile : 9869428528

Residence :
'Krishna'
G-37, Naraina Vihar
New Delhi - 110028
Phones 25799345
Telefax 011-25799345
Mobile 9811048330

Quote Ref No. ....
In your reply

To,
Dr. A. K. Saxena
B - 702, Sharmdeep CGHS Ltd.
Sector - 62, Noida (U.P.)

Sir,

You met me like a messiah when I was suffering from Disc Prolapse. Forty-five days of allopathic treatment gave me 30% relief whereafter you started treating me. You were candid enough to state that in case my body does not react positively within three days you will stop the treatment but fortunately this contingency did not arise. After 11 sittings I was near perfect and able to travel abroad where I walked a lot. But every science has its pros and cons. While allopathy cannot be discarded nonetheless acupressure as a science can be used to complement allopathic treatment and should not be considered as an alternative system as is commonly assumed I was impressed by your perfect diagnosis which matched my MRI reports. My experience motivates me to spread the good word about acupressure to one and all. I can offer no medical explanation for the miracle. My kudos to the miracle man who succeeded in effectively treating me.

With warm regards.

Yours Sincerely

(AJIT. S. BHAMSE)

Correspoindence at Delhi residence address only

Dr. SAVITA ANAND
I.F.S.
Principal Resident Commissioner

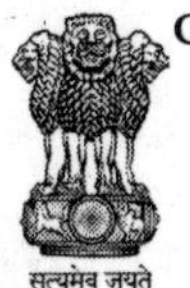

GOVERNMENT OF RAJASTHAN
Bikaner House, Pandara Road,
New Delhi-110011
Phone: 23381333
Fax.+91-11-23381802
E-mail: rcrajasthan@yahoo.com

MESSAGE

I have known Dr. A.K. Saxena for the last more than 20 years. During this period, I had undertaken acupressure treatment from him for my lower back. Recently, I developed cervical spondylosis along with severe vertigo. I had tremendous pain. I had taken allopathy treatment and also had MRI done. I was almost on bed for about two weeks. I had also taken physiotherapy sessions. Though there was improvement and I started feeling better, yet I was not comfortable and didn't feel confident about my recovery.

It was then I contacted Dr. A.K. Saxena for acupressure treatment. I wanted to show him my MRI but he mentioned that he would first give his diagnosis through pressing points and to my surprise, he could pin-point the exact vertebrae where I had problem and it matched with MRI also. He gave me four sittings and I felt very confident about my recovery and, in fact, I could resume office after two sittings.

Acupressure therapy is not only curative, it is preventive and diagnostic to a great extent. The expertise that Dr. Saxena has developed on this therapy is a God's gift to him and he uses his knowledge in providing relief to people and the best part is he voluntarily shares his knowledge with his patients so that after a few sittings, they are able to cure themselves. Besides, he also trains people who want to learn the nitty-gritty of this therapy.

I wish Dr. Saxena all the very best in life so that he continues to practise acupressure with zeal, fervour and passion.

1/8/2016

(Dr. Savita Anand)

Preface

Ever since the release of our third book on the subject, viz. *101 Q&A Acupressure and Reflexology* (English) in the year 2012 which was brought out to fulfill my quest to reach out to the people at the grassroot level and the long-awaited demand of my readers and students to bring out a book in question & answer form, incorporating the trigger points used by the practitioners of 'Acupuncture' and friends, from other streams of medical science, particularly some physiotherapists, who had adopted practicing 'acupressure', side by side, desired that I should share my experience(s) with them in the shape of "case studies", in a book form, so that the same could be used as a guide by prospective upcoming practitioners of this 'Art & Science' of Acupressure. Hindi translation of the aforesaid book was also brought out by the publishers in December 2014. The demand for bringing out the book incorporating Case Studies grew again.

Accordingly, the present book, *Handbook of Acupressure* is evolved. To share our experience(s), various cases have been incorporated in details. It gives details e.g. to give pressure on which trigger points, for how long, how many times, how many sessions, etc. Dietary regime/suggestions besides, Yoga tips (*Aasanas/Pranayam*), where necessary, have also been added to get even faster and long-term relief. I pen down my sincere gratitude to Dr. Preeti Pai, Yoga & Naturopathy Physician, Lady Hardinge Medical College & Hospital, New Delhi, whom I consider the best amongst the scores of Dieticians/Yoga & Naturopathy Physicians I have come across, for having agreed to co-author this book and provide detailed disease specific diet charts as well as Yoga tips, which shall go a long way in prevention as well as cure to the readers who imbibe these means in their life-style.

I would like to reiterate that going by the established norm that the prime concern of the patient is to get relief from pain and disease, whereas we advocate co-management, i.e. taking treatment using acupressure technique as a home remedy side by side while taking treatment in either of the conventional streams of medicine, of the choice of the patient depending upon the seriousness of the ailment. What should never be allowed to lose sight off is that the treatment should always be preceded by proper diagnosis at the hands of a physician, so as to ensure that in case(s) where vital organs of the body, e.g. heart, kidney, liver, etc. are involved, the symptoms might not get overlooked and on a later date disease of more serious nature raise its head. However, in case(s) of day-to-day ailments, e.g. back/knee/heel pains; cervical spondylosis; migraine; insomnia; indigestion; constipation; piles, etc., where apparently there is no immediate risk to life, a fair trial to non-conventional stream of treatment, e.g. diet regulation, Yoga, acupressure should be banked upon. As a word of caution, in case enough relief is not felt within a week, the patient should opt for other modes of treatment.

With all humility, we invite positive suggestions/criticism towards further improvement so that our effort is put to the best use for benefit of suffering mankind for the times to come.

— Dr. A.K. Saxena

Introduction

There can be no second opinion about the fact that modern medicine has greatly contributed towards the improvement of health care, thereby increasing the life span. But in the process science took precedence and administration of medicines became mechanical, as life was unfortunately looked at as a purely chemical phenomenon. Practitioners of modern medicine regarded human body more or less as a machine, made up of complex collection of parts. Ancient natural medical practices were pushed into the background or frequently suppressed.

However, several decades down the time-line, disillusionment with modern medicines as a panacea, has resulted into resurgence and demand for natural form of therapies. Realization has dawned upon the people that each of the conventional and non-conventional practices has their role in healthcare and that ideally these should work together. It has been realized that a holistic approach has to be taken and health care aspect handled by taking care of not only 'body' but that of 'mind' (emotional aspect), and of 'soul' (spiritual aspect) too.

One of the World Health Organization reports reads:

"For too long traditional systems of medicine and 'modern' medicine have gone their separate ways in mutual antipathy. Yet are not their goals identical – to improve the health of mankind and thereby the quality of life? Only the blinkered mind would assume that each has nothing to do with the other."

Human body possesses immense natural strength to heal itself from most of the diseases. What is required is to tap this natural energy to rejuvenate it. Growing consciousness about the side effect of the medicine and the exorbitant cost factor has perhaps led to the emergence of so many 'Alternative Therapies'. A few of these being Zone therapy, Magnet therapy, Hydro therapy, Color therapy, Aroma therapy, etc., besides Ancient Indian Science of 'Yoga & Naturopathy' coming back with a bang and getting recognition at the international level, thanks to the interest and effort of our Hon'ble Prime Minister Mr. Narendra Modi. Besides, Acupressure, an improvised version of the 'Ancient Science' called "Acupuncture" has of late, gained lot of prominence over the recent decades and has emerged as one of the most sought-after systems that are capable of reviving and revitalizing the hidden curative powers within our bodies. Moreover, it is non-conventional and non-interventional besides being simple to perform, usable as a home remedy and without fear of any side effect because no medicine in any form has to be administered. All the more it is totally non-invasive.

In this context, we shall be failing in our duty, in case we don't clarify, that we prefer to call all the aforesaid therapies as "Complementary Therapies" and 'not' "Alternative Therapies", as the term 'Alternative' improperly communicates, as if an alternative to the conventional medicine is being provided. It smacks of unacceptability, whereas there is no such attempt whatsoever. The ultimate goal of all of us, i.e. the patient, the physician or surgeon or the practitioner of the non-conventional (complementary) therapy, is to achieve a state of health/well-being at the earliest, irrespective of how and by what means it is achieved. It is heartening to note that the practitioners of medicine and complementary therapies have started joining hands to work together for the benefit of patients. With more practitioners of medicine qualifying in complementary therapies, they have started laying emphasis on body, mind, and soul; eating for health and vitality, awareness about exercise and self-help measures to enhance and improve physical, emotional and spiritual health, and well-being.

One is in good health when the flow of energy (the vital force) through the meridians of the body is smooth, balanced and unobstructed. The moment this flow is adversely affected, it may result in pain or disease. Stomach disorders, colds, allergies or fatigue are the warning signals given by our body to alert that the flow of vital force is disturbed or blocked. In case one does not take a timely note of these warning signals to take corrective steps, serious ailments may occur. By learning to apply gentle pressure on certain key pressure points with one's thumb or finger tips, these imbalances can be corrected to restore good health and overcome pain.

Acupressure is capable of regulating various systems in our body, including nervous and circulatory systems. Increasing circulation helps in flushing out the toxins from the body and bringing in nutrients and oxygen to cells. It also triggers the brain to release a chemical called 'endorphin', which is a natural pain killer and capable of bringing a feeling of well-being in our body. When pressure is given at various pressure (reflex) points, pertaining to various organs, while treating a patient, toxins, calcium, urea etc., deposited in crystalline form at the nerve endings in the soles and the palms gets crushed and thrown out of the body from different outlets. In this manner, acupressure has been found to be one of the simplest and most effective methods of healing and restoring normal functioning of the body in a natural way. Acupressure cleanses the body of toxins and impurities which accumulate at the nerve endings leading to many ailments. These toxins obstruct the normal flow of energy to various organs thereby disturbing the balance of whole body.

My experience of over 25 years with various patients, reveals that the results attained through application of "Acupressure–Reflexology" technique are very encouraging, not only in helping out patients suffering from common ailments, e.g. cervical/lumber spondylosis; sinusitis; backaches; knee/heel pains; sciatica; prolapsed disc; piles; I.B.S.; P.M.S.; C.T.S.; insomnia; depression; asthma; hypertension; fits; ulcers; tennis elbow, etc., but also, at times it has been found to be of immense help in providing almost complete cure to the critically ill patients, following the co-management concept. Needless to say that a lot depends on the willpower, body response and of course faith of the patient in the therapy as well as in the therapist. The Body-Mind connection hold so true!

What encourages us further in our resolve to take this 'Art & Science' to the grassroot level is the growing number of its admirers in the most sought-after stream of Medical Science– "Allopathy". Even senior allopathic physician and surgeons have been recommending patients to take Acupressure treatment while continuing to take treatment in conventional stream. The results too are highly encouraging. Our resolve further strengthens when practicing medicos/ physiotherapists approach me for 'Training' in Acupressure at our Centre.

Our sincere advice to our students as well as to the readers of our book(s), is that "The therapy is fool proof and in case you do not get the results to the desired extent, blame the therapist not the therapy". Be honest, give a second thought to find out (re-access–assess) where we went wrong, not to give up, and try again, as sooner or later the body will favourably respond.

□

Foreword

Many natural forms of therapies have emerged in the recent past, like Acupressure/Reflexology, Zone therapy, Reiki, Shiatsu, Color therapy, Magnet therapy, Hydro therapy, etc. Among these, Acupressure holds pride of place for its effectiveness, simplicity, and adaptability to self-care. It is totally non-interventional, non-invasive and all the more not only curative, but preventive as well. It was derived from an age-old therapy called 'Acupuncture', which is almost 5,000 years old. Both Acupuncture and Acupressure are based on Reflexology, and in fact, Acupressure is an improvised form of Acupuncture, to make it easier to practice, so that it can be used as a home remedy as no medication/incision is required. All that it requires is to use the healing power of human body itself to overcome the imbalances in the chemicals energy levels, within the meridians in the body. This is accomplished by applying pressure over the reflex points corresponding to various organs of body, which are located in the soles and the palms. A disease is the outcome of the imbalances caused by certain bottlenecks that impede smooth flow of vital chemicals and forces in the body. Once these bottlenecks are removed, the normal state of health is restored.

Reflexology is a fascinating science that has created a niche in the field of alternative medicine, being based on the physiological as well as neurological scientific factors. Skills of an expert practitioner add further value to it.

Acupressure is a technique, in which pressure is given over specific reflex points over the feet and is based on the premise that reflex areas on the feet correspond to all organs, glands, vital points of the body. The same can be achieved from palm/ears too. However, it can be done with ease over the feet where it is easier to locate the reflex points, the size of a feet being large.

There can be no doubt that modern medicine has contributed greatly towards the improvement of health care, for instance, handling of a complicated surgery is a notable contribution of modern science. But need of the times is that both modern and alternative streams help better to cure the patients. The best way, perhaps, would be that both supplement their roles and work together for the benefit of all.

In the line of above, I am highly impressed by the approach of the authors and their vision. They have tried to bring around this point and gone a step further by coining the word 'co-management' in place of 'alternate medicine', the former adequately recognizing co-operation between the streams to enjoy bliss of their confluence.

The authors, Dr. A.K. Saxena and Dr. (Mrs.) Preeti Pai, have brought out their rich and long experience, in a 'Capsule' form in this book for the benefit of readers, prospective practitioners. It is ably supported with figures to pin point the precise location of the pressure points. They have also effectively elaborated about the symptoms encountered in each case and given pressure points to achieve amazing results, for even successfully 'co-managing' certain dreaded diseases. Moreover, dietary and Yoga tips have been aptly added for faster and lasting recovery.

The authors, Dr. A.K. Saxena and Dr. (Mrs.) Preeti Pai are accomplished writers, between them having authored valuable books like (i) *Miraculous Effects of Acupressure* (English and Marathi with its e-book being brought out), Bengali (under print) and Assamese (under print); (ii) *Acupressure aur Swasth Jeevan* Hindi and Gujarati; (iii) *101 Q*

& A Acupressure & Reflexology (English, Hindi with Bengali under print). They have also ceaselessly imparted effective training for more than a dozen of years, having successfully trained more than 200 persons from all walks of life. They have also been attending patients in the hospitals of repute on call.

I am sure that all stakeholders would find this book immensely valuable and utilize it frequently.

— Dr. P.K. Anand, IAS (retd.),
Senior Consultant, NITI Aayog,
(Former Senior Adviser, Planning Commission)

Contents

Case–1
CAD, Multiple Organ Failure

This was in the year 2006 I attended a 45 years old gentleman, Mr. Z, well built, tall, weight around 100 kg, with critical coronary artery disease, admitted in the CCU of a hospital of international repute in Delhi, who had developed a cardiac arrest post angiography and was taken up for emergency bypass surgery while continuing CPR. Post surgery, the patient developed signs of severe Hypoxic encephalopathy and critical illness myoneuropathy. He was comatose and could not move either of his limbs. MRI Scan suggested poor prognosis.

Thanks to the open mindedness of the doctors attending on him that at such a stage they thought of co-managing the case, while continuing the treatment conventionally. I was called and, in a brief meeting, I was informed about the status of the patient's condition. Although the condition of the patient was really critical with high grade fever, acute septicemia, multi organ failure, on dialysis thrice a week, going by the resolve "never give up", I accepted the case. Started giving pressure over the trigger points pertaining to the neuro as well as nervous system and the pressure points pertaining to voice specifically, as shown by the shaded portion over the inner edges of the big toes and the thumbs, to begin with. Besides, I also gave pressure over the primary pressure points pertaining to the vitals, e.g. brain, heart, liver, kidneys, etc. as have been shown in the diagrams. Besides above, the following pressure points

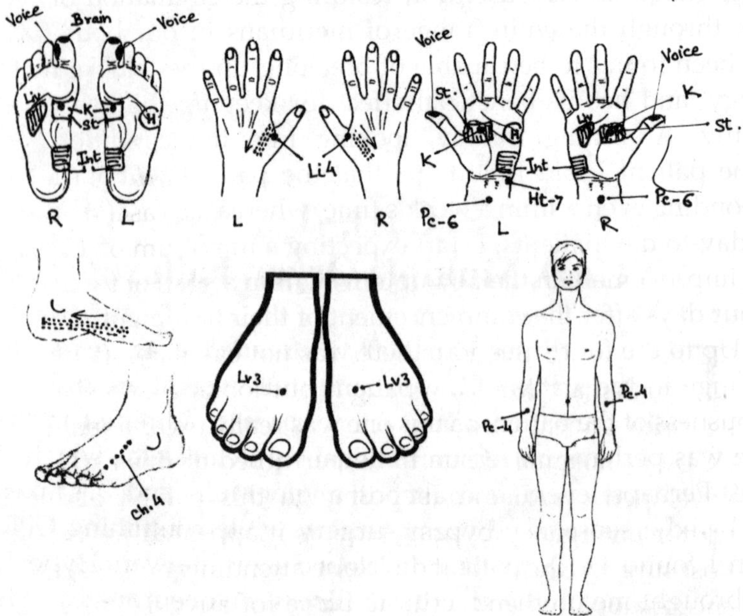

were also stimulated on a daily basis : Ht-7 (The Mind Door) was pressed as this is the source point to stimulate the heart meridian. It not only nourishes the heart but also helps in soothing the emotions and calming the mind. Its location has been depicted in the figure. Next point was Pc-6, it has been named according to its potential and as such is known as 'Heart Protector'. Has been found to be of immense use in over coming any sort of discomfort or pain in the heart region. It also restores the flow of Ch'i and blood in the heart region. This point is located two thumb widths above the wrist crease in the middle of the arm on the palm side of the wrist as shown in the figure.

Next set of points pressed were Pc-4, 'The Cleft Gate' as this point is known for its ability to overcome any sort of discomfort in the chest area. In case(s) where discomfort or pain in the chest area is intense, this point should be pressed on both the arms first of all. To complete the session, gave pressure over Li-4 and Lv-3. This combination known as

"Four Gates" is very useful in restoring the circulation of Ch'i, through the entire range of meridians in our body. Has been found to be capable of breaking up the 'blocked energy' and has its beneficial effect for keeping the heart healthy. Admitting frankly, looking into the condition of the patient I had little hope that the patient will start responding even within a week's time, whereas in case(s) of my day-to-day patients, I start expecting a minimum of 10-15% improvement in their symptoms within a span of three to four days after the commencement of their treatment.

Up to the fourth session, there was not even an iota of a change in the status of the patient but looking into the seriousness of the patient as this one was really exceptional, there was perhaps no reason to be perturbed at this early stage. Perhaps, every one attending on this patient had developed a sense of belongingness, as it appeared to me when I found Dr. X, the Cardiologist attending him who had brought me on the scene, had come for a round early morning, all the way from his home, which was around six kms apart, and was returning home, at 7.00 am, when I was climbing the stairs in the hospital to attend the patient. He stopped me and remarked, "Congrats, doc, your patient has started responding". I was taken aback and told the doctor, "Are you kidding? Only last night when I went back around 10.15 pm after attending him, there was no change in his status?" He said, "please go and check yourself". When I entered the CTVS, ICU, in the hospital, wife of the patient, who had been allowed to be with the patient all the time as a special case, tried to touch my feet. When stopped by me, she exclaimed, Sir, he has started responding! As I wanted to check for myself, I touched his brain point and the patient who used to lie in bed like a pumpkin and was not able to even close his eyes, closed his eyes in token of having felt the sensation of 'pain'. I wanted to further confirm whether his other faculties were also responding, I pressed on a pressure point which was not supposed to react and he did not react.

Then I addressed him by his name and asked him to close his eyes in case it hurts (the patient was not able to speak as he had lost his voice). When I pressed the trigger point pertaining to the brain and the "Liv-3", without informing him, he closed his eyes that exhibited signs of sensation of 'pain'.

Encouraged by the response, I added the pressure points for the stimulation of the digestive and other systems, as has been shown. By the time 08-10 sessions were completed, the patient started moving his limbs on demand though with some amount of effort and started speaking too. The number of three dialysis per week was also reduced to two in a week, ventilator support was also withdrawn. It took around 25 sessions for the total recovery, the patient was discharged and had been doing well on follow ups in the hospital, had resumed work.

Personally, I would like to give the entire credit to Dr. X, the Senior Consultant, Interventional Cardiologist, of the hospital, whose open mindedness and broad thinking led to the miraculous recovery of the patient by virtue of co-management of the case. Since then many other Sr. Cardiologists from the same hospital, started associating me in co-managing similar critically ill cases and have been occasionally associating me in the co-management of critical cases and the success rate has fortunately been pretty encouraging.

□

Case–2
Kidney Failure

In case I can recall correctly, this case was dealt with in the year 1995. A gentleman aged around 39 years called me over phone to say that I am Mr. A, aged 39 years have been suffering for more than five years due to 'Kidney' problem, had been undergoing treatment in a hospital of high repute in Delhi. Now they have told me to go for at least one Kidney transplant within three months or so since both my kidneys have almost failed, the reported loss was 80% and 85%. When I told him to follow the doctors advice, he stated that he was not in a position to bear the cost. Truly speaking, I was not so confident about my own capability to handle such a critical case, with merely 5-6 years of experience. I told him to go for some other treatment and see some good 'Homeopath' since I personally have great faith in Homeopathy. But the patient insisted that he wanted to come to me only, since despite my telling him that in the given circumstances, when the damage to both the kidneys is so high, what a naturopath of my stature can do for you, he retorted that the person who has referred me to you has already told me that you will not be ready to take my case but he has also told me that you may be of help, as such he has decided to take treatment from me at his risk.

The patient came with his wife at the appointed time, along with his papers. After going through his reports wherein the parameters were obviously found to be very high, S.Cretanine was 9.7. However, to my utter surprise,

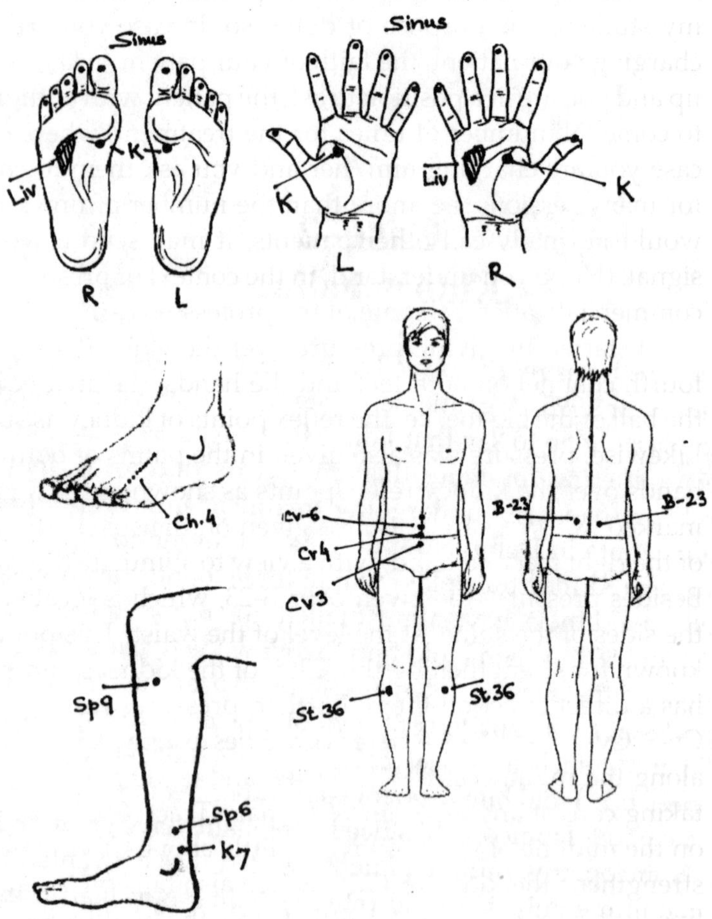

the general condition of the patient was not as bad as any one would have imagined based on the extent of damage reported over phone. There was not much edema over the body/legs/feet, though the muscles of both the legs were extremely week. The treatment commenced, though reluctantly, but looking into their faith, I could not say no to them. (But I decided not to charge them. This I do with most of the serious/critical cases, where I myself am not sure about the recovery of the patient, for my own satisfaction.

Here I want to take this opportunity to convey to my students the purpose of doing so. In case you are not charging your patient, the faith of your patient further goes up and you are in a position to ask the patient with authority to come 'N' number of times for the treatment, whereas in case you are charging him/her and you ask them to come for many sessions, i.e. more than the number of times you would normally call other patients, it may send a wrong signal. (Hope you understand, in the context of present-day commercialization by some of the professionals.)

I started by giving pressure over the Sinus Points; the fourth channel on both feet and the hands; the area below the ball of the big toe, i.e. the reflex points of kidney as such. Likewise, pressure was also given in the palms of both the hands over the kidney reflex points as shown in the figure, marked 'K'. Pressure was also given on the sole and palm of the right feet and hand, with a view to stimulate the liver. Besides pressure was given over B-23, which is located on the sides of the spine, at the level of the waist. This point is known for strengthening the 'Ch'i' of the kidneys and thus has a direct effect on them. Further, pressure was given at Cv-3, Cv-4, and Cv-6, whereas Cv-3 lies exactly at the centre along the midline of the abdomen and is very effective in taking care of any disorder of Urinary Tract, Cv-4 also lies on the midline of the abdomen, a little above Cv-3, this too strengthens the kidneys. Cv-6 which also falls on the same line little above Cv-4 and a little below the 'umbilicus' also strengthens the kidneys. In addition pressure was given over Sp-6; St-36; Sp-9 and Kd-7. Whereas Sp-6, known as "three yin meeting point" strengthens three meridians, viz. kidney, liver, and spleen at the same time, located four finger width above the ankle bone and is considered to be one of the most important pressure points while healing a patient suffering from kidney, liver or spleen problem, St-36 when used in combination with Sp-6 strengthens the whole body, tones the muscles and revitalizes the entire body. Sp-9 lies on the inside of the leg, under the shin bone and giving pressure on this point helps in reducing edema, water retention by regulating the water metabolism in our body. Giving pressure on Kd-7 takes care of the Yang aspect of kidney's Ch'i. For the sake of convenience, these pressure points have been marked in figure.

By the time, around 10 sessions or so were over, the patient started showing substantial signs of improvement. Muscle strength in his lower limbs improved beyond expectation, the patient started having a feeling of wellness, his confidence level exhibited a marked change, his wife informed that she has noticed definite change in his appetite, he was able to get far better sleep. I asked the patient not to come every day anymore but to come on alternate days, but the patient insisted for every day visit. Some how I could convince him that daily sessions were no more required since he was himself feeling better and despite not going for dialysis more than once in the previous week, his S. Cretanine level had come down to 5.4.

During the above said period, I always made sure that the patient was under regular supervision of his physician and taking the treatment he was getting before coming to me to ensure that things may not go from bad to worse in case acupressure treatment does not suit him since the ailment the patient had been suffering could have been life threatening as well. In all, I might have given him around 20 to 25 sessions and by that time the patient had totally recovered, dialysis was stopped and he resumed work. The patient had been doing well on follow-ups, as reported about four years ago.

□

Case–3
Water Retention/UTI

A female patient Ms. Z, aged about 32 years, daughter of a very Senior Police Officer from Himachal Pradesh, tall and well built, working in an MNC in a pretty senior position, was brought to my clinic with "water retention problem". Her entire body was 'bloated', she was not in a position to pass urine. She informed me that she had been depending on an allopathic drug, "Lassix" and despite taking 40 mg dose of the above said medicine every day, she could pass urine in "drops"only. This was hampering her day to day activity and her overall health badly effected. Clearly, the case indicated 'kidney malfunctioning'.

Started with giving pressure over the reflex points of kidneys followed by giving pressure over the reflex area for the urinary bladder on both soles and palms, as indicated. These pressure points have a direct bearing, as point K nourishes the kidneys, whereas point B stimulates the 'urinary bladder'. After having given pressure over these reflexes, pressure needs to be given on the shaded area over the wrists of both the hands, the points marked thereon. These points represent the genitals and stimulating them has been found to be of immense benefit in overcoming 'urinary problems', these points have also been found to be much beneficial in overcoming 'UTI' problem. It would be even better in case pressure as indicated above is given on both sides of the wrist, after stimulating the shaded area on the wrist by giving massage like pressure in the indicated

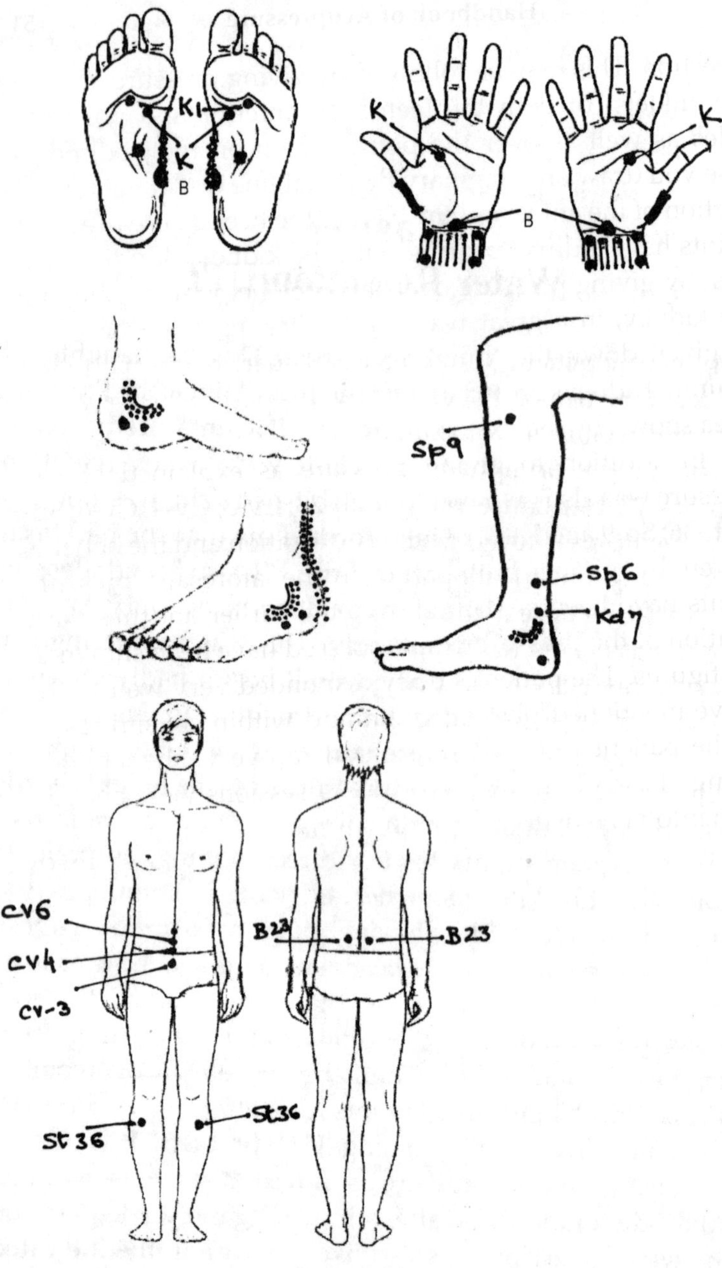
K1
K
B
K
K
B
Sp9
Sp6
Kd7
CV6
CV4
CV-3
B23
B23
St36
St 36

direction. This may be followed by giving pressure around the ankle(s) of both the feet, both anterior and posterior sides as well as over the point shown on the midline in case you draw an imaginary diagonal line down the lowest portion of the ankle and the base of the heel. These pressure points have a direct bearing with the kidney meridian and thereby giving pressure over this area helps strengthening the kidney, in a great way. Thereafter, pressure needs to be given down the 'Lumbo-Saccral' part of the vertebral column. Kidneys are nourished by this part of the vertebrae (area shown by the xxxxxx lines).

In addition to giving pressure as explained above, pressure was also given on Kd-1; B-23; Cv-3; Cv-4; Cv-6; Sp-6; St.-36; Sp-9 and Kd-7 points. The location and the benefits driven by giving pressure over the aforesaid pressure points have been explained in detail earlier and the exact location of the pressure points pressed have been shown in the figures. The patient's body responded very well to the above-mentioned plan of action and within six sittings or so the patient reported substantial recovery, she stopped taking "Lassix". In all around 13-14 sessions were enough for her total recovery.

□

Case–4
Prolapse Disc

Mr. A, aged about 50 years, a tall and healthy gentleman, a senior advocate in the Supreme Court, on being refered to me by an old patient of mine, came with prolapse disc problem in the year 2005. He had been advised surgery at the earliest. Whereas, like any other patient he wanted to avoid surgery since the success rate is not reportedly too high as compared to the hassle of undergoing surgery, confinement to bed, etc., and for a professional of his stature it was a little more of a problem. Yet another problem he was facing was that he had to travel to USA to join his son after barely 11 days. He wanted me to commit that he would be able to travel.

On examination, I found that as in most of such cases, the problem was at "L-4, L-5 and S-1" level, besides the Sciatic nerve was getting pressed. I told the patient in very clear terms that it would be highly improper for me to make any commitment at that stage, as to whether he would be able to travel after 10-11 days, as it would solely depend how his body reacts to this treatment. As such, I told him to wait and watch for his body response to the treatment for about 3-4 sessions, before taking a decision on his travel plans. Since he had to travel a lot to reach me, he was facing some problem but he insisted on continuing the treatment, in the hope that he would be able to avoid surgery and travel as scheduled.

I started his treatment with the following action plan: Began with stimulating the Lumbo-Sacral region over the

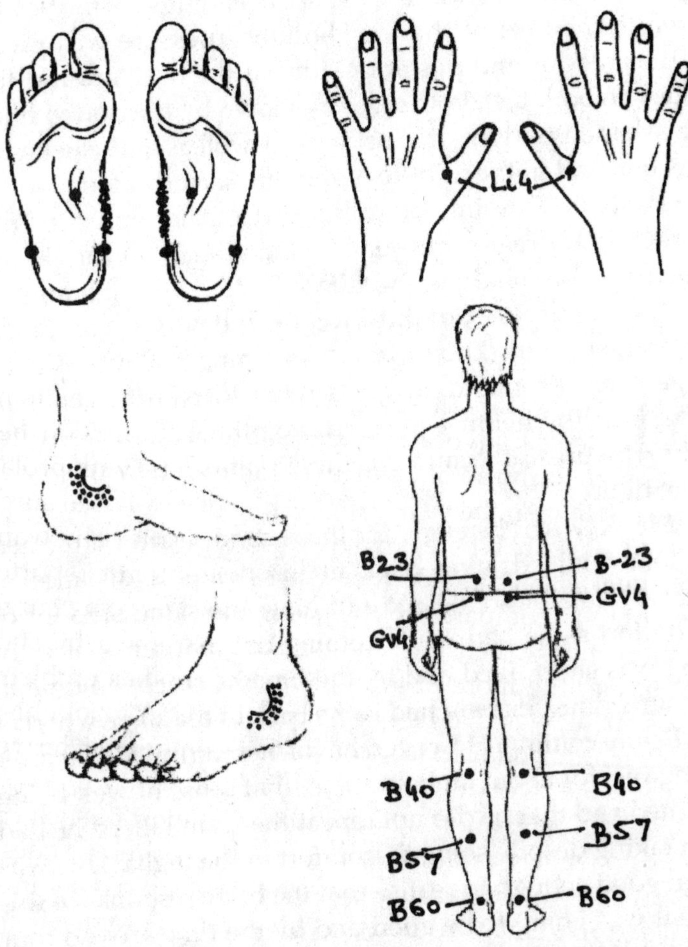

soles and the palms. Direct pressure was given on the areas marked "xxxxxx" on the Lumbo-Sacral part for about 30 seconds over each reflex point as shown in the figure, since giving pressure over a single reflex point for 30 seconds would have certainly made the area tender to the pressure, this was done in the fractions of eight to ten seconds in one go on every point thus giving pressure on one point three to four times in one session. This was followed by giving pressure over the other trigger points marked in the figure, referred to above. These are the nerve endings for the Sciatic nerve in the heel of the feet. Besides, pressure was given on the anterior and posterior sides of the heel, around the ankles on both feet, both sides as shown by the dotted lines – the shaded portion- in clockwise as well as anti-clockwise direction and in the middle of the sole, as indicated.

Patients suffering from any sort of discomfort in the Lumbo-Sacral region respond tremendously to the points which fall on bladder meridian (B-23); B-40 (command point) — on the back of the knee; B-57; B-60; Cv-4 and Li-4, this trigger point (known as — adjoining valley) over the Large Intestine meridian gives relief to pain in any part of the body by helping in circulating the Ch'i in the entire body. The precise location of these points has been shown in the figure.

Mr. A, when he came for the second session informed me that while driving back to his home, a distance of about 40 kms or so, he did not have the same amount of discomfort as he had while coming but that sense of well-being was short lived and by the time he reached home in an hour's time, his pain had come back to the stage where it was before coming. However, he further informed that after taking rest for about an hour or so, that sense of well-being returned and that he did not repeat the 'pain killers' he had been taking despite some discomfort in the night. That was a sign good enough to realise that the body response of this patient was going to be good and by the time around four sessions were completed, the patient reported 15 to 20% recovery. He had to take pain killer only once in this span of four days. This was a good news to both of us. He was very hopeful that he would be able to travel, however, I still told him to hold taking a final decision for yet another three to four sessions. By the time seven sessions were completed, he reported around 50% recovery and at that stage, I too gave him a nod that he may travel.

Just to check, how his body responds in case a session

is skipped, I told him to give a gap of a day, but he was not willing for it. Some how I could convince him to my plan and fortunately there was no going back by giving a break in the sitting/session. In all I gave him 10 sessions and the target was accomplished, Mr. A, travelled to the States and to add to my happiness he telephoned from New York that he was fine and was able to move about freely. As a precaution, I had advised him not to over exert, cautiously handle his luggage and given him a chart of the pressure points to be pressed in the event pain recurs and a probe to press those point, but when he came back he reported that during his entire stay of around 20 days there, he had to ask his son only two times to give him pressure over the prescribed points and he had no problem whatsoever. After he came back home, he wrote a letter of thanks to me as a token of his gratitude.

Based on this case and my experience in hundreds of similar other cases, I would like to share with my readers that in a good number of cases recovery comes sooner or later, either fully or partially. Case history of some more case(s) of this type shall be discussed ahead which were having some other associated problems too and were handled successfully.

□

Case–5
Tennis Elbow

Mr. K, an IPS (retd.), a well-built gentleman of about 64 yrs., approached me for his 'Tennis Elbow' pain which he had been suffering for more than 5-6 years. He admitted that he had come to me on the recommendation of some colleague, to try out this stream of treatment also, after having undergone treatment at many outlets of repute since according to him best of medical care was available to him by virtue of his position, but unfortunately he did not get relief at all or at places he got partial relief only which recurred shortly after the treatment was stopped.

I commenced the treatment by giving pressure over the reflex area of the 'Sinus points' as shown in figure, followed by giving pressure over other point as shown. This point can be located by closing your fist and lies where the middle finger touches the palm. Although it hurts badly on being pressed, this has been found to be highly beneficial in over coming pain in the front part of the arm. Give moderate pressure only so that the point does not become very tender to touch. Also in case pressure is given over the points marked in the fore arm, it gives tremendous help in overcoming 'Tennis Elbow' problem. Thereafter pressed Li-4, which is located in the wedge between the thumb and the index finger. Followed by this was Li-11, a pressure point that falls over the crease when we fold our forearm to touch our shoulder. These points are highly beneficial in overcoming pain in the arm, shoulder and of course the

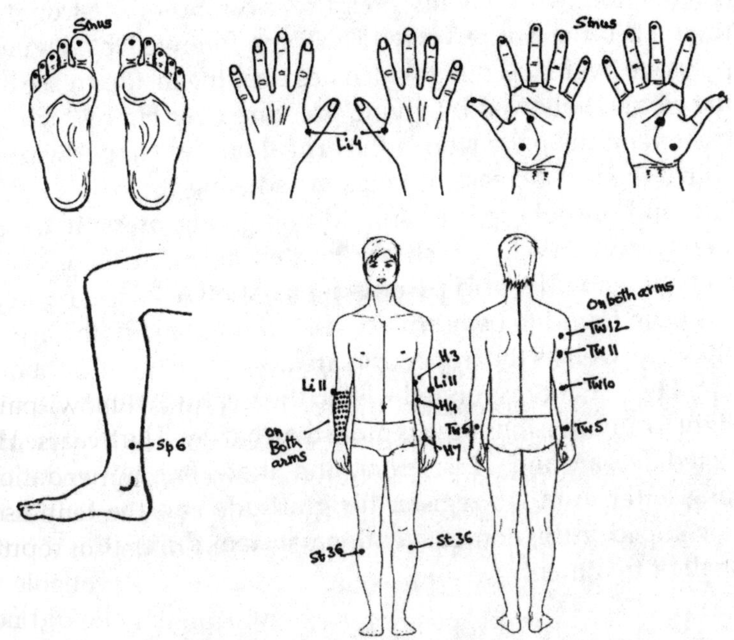

elbow. This was followed by giving pressure over the Triple Warmer point Nos. 5, 10, 11 and 12, followed by St-36 given in conjunction with Sp-6, Ht-3, Ht.-4, and Ht-7. TW-5 (Outer Gate) is located mid way between the ulna and radius about three finger width above the wrist crease towards the elbow bone on the outside of the wrist (back side). The triple warmer channel runs up the back of the arm to the shoulder and neck, then moves around to the side of the neck. This point is very useful to treat any problem with the arm, up to shoulder and neck. Next gave pressure on TW-10 (Heavenly well) which is located one thumb width above the tip of elbow, towards the shoulder. It helps relieve the elbow pain, stiffness of the elbow, and the shoulder. Deep breathing simultaneously shall further improve its effect over this area. Thereafter, give pressure on St-36 which lies four finger widths below the kneecap, this point strengthens the whole body, tones up the muscles and when given in conjunction with giving pressure over Sp-6, it strongly revitalizes the entire body. This was followed by giving pressure over Ht-3 point which lies over the inside crease of the elbow. Followed by giving pressure over Ht-4 which is located on the palm side of the arm about two finger width above the wrist crease. It helps in reducing the pain in the arm and 'muscle spasm'. In addition giving pressure over TW-11 and TW-12 which are located between the elbow and the shoulder triceps muscle, as shown in the figure, has been found to be useful in overcoming pain in the arm, elbow as well as the upper arm area.

The patient responded well to the treatment and within eight to nine sessions he was more than happy. The treatment lasted for around 12 sessions and thereafter he wrote a long letter to me to register his gratitude and the faith he developed, in this non-conventional system, during this short spell of treatment.

□

Case–6
Knee Problem

Mr. K, whose case has been discussed above was so much overwhelmed by his treatment and consequent recovery, since he had gone from pillar to post for the treatment of his 'Tennis Elbow' without much success, that he returned with his wife Mrs. K for the treatment of her 'knee pain', from which she had been suffering a lot and had been advised 'surgery' at the earliest by as many as 2-3 orthopedic surgeons. Discussions with Mrs. K, revealed that she has been very active throughout her life, engaging herself in lots of social activities as well as 'welfare activities' for the staff members in the force, at the grassroot level, her husband being a very senior police officer. Both husband and wife were very fond of their long morning walks But due to her knee pain, her entire lifestyle had come to a standstill.

One thing very positive, I noticed with the patient was that owing to her lifestyle, her body weight was commensurate to her height, her willpower was strong and above all she was very keen to overcome the problem at its earliest and in the process, was willing to abide by any restrictions prescribed and come regularly for the treatment, encouraged by the results they got in her husband's treatment. The treatment commenced and I told them that for four to five sessions they should not expect any miracles and in case her body responds then only we will continue with her treatment. I started with giving

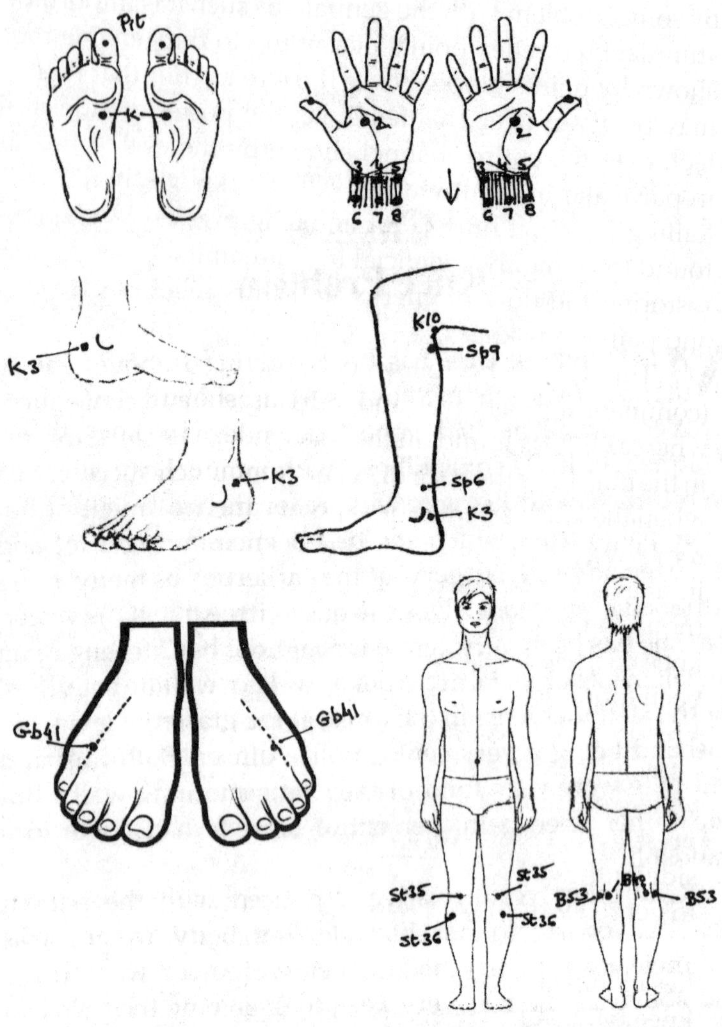

pressure over point pertaining to the 'pituitary' and kidneys point, for the reason that whereas stimulating pituitary gland point improves the functioning of all the endocrine glands, strengthening of kidneys helps in throwing out unwanted accumulations in our body. After doing this on both the soles and the palms respectively. At times it has been observed that knee and Lower back pains are caused by some problem with the genitals, as such it is important to stimulate the reflex points pertaining to the genitals too as shown by points marked over the wrist. After that pressure may be given over channel 4, i.e. the posterior side of the feet, over the entire channel shown by the dotted line and in particular at point marked 'Gb-41' (known by the name 'falling tears'), it hurts a lot on being pressed but has been found to be highly beneficial in overcoming 'knee pain', by restoring the flow of energy and thus relieves discomfort and pain in the knees.

This has to be followed by giving pressure on B-53 (commanding activity) and B-54 as shown in the figure, whereas B-53 is found on the outer side of the knee, B-40 lies in the middle of the back of knee, over the crease that is found when the knee is bent. These points are highly beneficial for removing stiffness and pain in the knees. B-40 is also usefull in alleviating 'sciatica pain'. Then give pressure on 'K-10' (nourishing valley), which lies on the inner edge of the knee crease, in the hollow between the two tendons and has been found to be highly effective in overcoming knee pain. Pressing 'Sp-9', which lies inside on the leg under the shin bone, just below the bulge, helps in reducing the edema, water retention and other discomfort in the knee area. Also press Lv-8 (crooked spring), which is located over the inner side of the knee, where the crease ends when knee is bent, to get relief from pain and swelling in the knees. Also press 'K-3'; St-35 and St-36 as shown in the figure. Whereas St-35 lies in the outer indentation below the knee cap and relieves knee pain; stiffness and edema, St-36 which lies four finger widths below the knee cap, one finger width on the outside of the shin bone, is known to strengthen the whole body, tones up the muscles, particularly when used in conjunction with Sp-6, it strongly revitalizes the whole body.

Fortunately, by the time three sessions of the treatment were over, Mrs. K started to have a sense of well being, so much so that she went for a 3 km walk on the fourth day morning, which slightly aggravated discomfort in one of her knees. When she came for the session in the evening that day, she reported that the discomfort in her knee has reversed by around 30%. On probing she informed that she had gone for a long walk in the morning. She was advised that she should gradually put her knee to stress and should not try to over do even after the treatment was over. The very next day when she came back for the session she reported that her discomfort has gone and she did go for the morning walk but as per my advise, rested for a while the moment she felt stress in the knee area and after taking rest for 2-3 minutes she restarted without any aggravation. The treatment lasted for about 14-15 sessions in all. She had been in touch with me, ever thankful for being able to avert surgery which was being considered to be imminent. Could restart her morning walks. This fact her husband later confirmed to me through a letter.

□

Case–7

Peptic Ulcer and Other Associated Probs

Some time in the year 1995, an old school-time friend of mine telephoned me to inform that his father was having a very bad time with severe symptoms of indigestion; heartburn, lack of appetite pain in the abdomen associated with nausea and vomiting. The diagnosis was reported to be 'Peptic Ulcers', as per the doctor attending the patient. He further informed me that since his father has had lot of allopathic medicines in the past, he has developed a sort of aversion towards allopathic medicines and as such he has taken appointment with one of the best-known Homeopaths in Delhi (Dr. Jugal Kishore), but the appointment is after four days and in the meanwhile, he inquired, in case I can help his father in this condition. I told him that there was no harm in giving acupressure therapy in case his father was willing, only constraint I told him was that I will be able to attend him late in the evening say around 9.30 pm or so in view of my previous appointments. He called back to inform that his father was more than willing and said that he would bring his father to my home, which I did not consider to be proper, looking into the condition of the patient and our close friendship.

I visited him at the appointed time and found the patient to be eagerly waiting, the first positive sign from the point of view of a Naturopath that the patient should have faith in the therapy as also the therapist. Since the patient was working as a private secretary to a senior officer, about

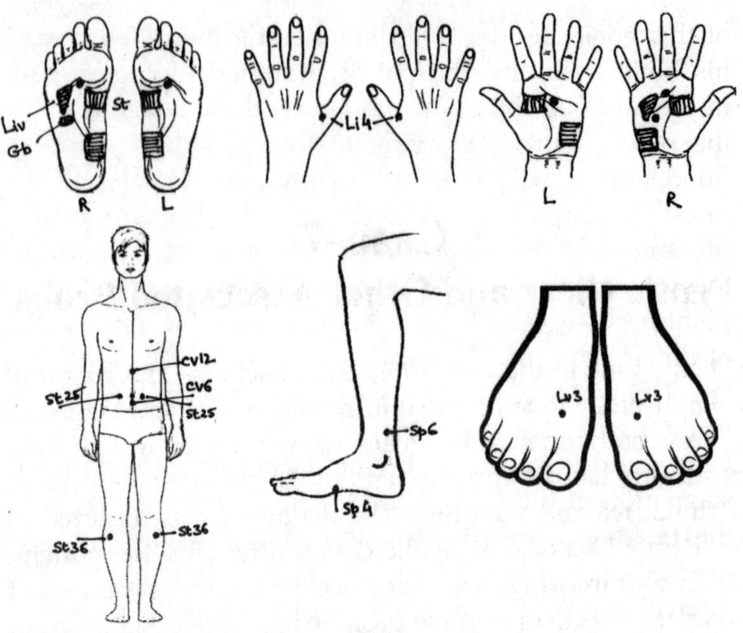

whose temper/way of working , he used to discuss with me whenever I happened to visit their house. I could guess that one of the prime causes of the severe heartburn he has been experiencing could be the stress factor and tension at workplace. Besides, I knew the patient temperamentally. He was always in a hurry, not devoting enough time while eating and not having very sound eating habits. Very fond of eating fried food, at times also stale food, just gulping his food in a hurry without allowing proper time to chew.

After reassuring the patient that soon he will be under the care of one of the best Homeopaths of his choice and that hopefully my treatment will also get him some respite, I commenced his treatment after taking assurance from him that he will strictly follow the advice I was going to give about his food intake. As a matter of fact, he was not able to consume any thing since he was vomiting whatever he was consuming. I told him to start taking diet according to the diet chart prescribed for him, added in the later part of this book. Besides, after stimulating the reflex areas in his both soles and the palms, I started giving pressure in the areas as shown in the figure, these areas belong to the reflex points pertaining to liver, stomach, pancreas, duodenum, gall bladder diaphragm (solar plexus), intestines (large and small) respectively. Thereafter I gave pressure on Liv-3, which lies between the big and second toes on top of the foot. The importance of pressing this point needs no emphasis. It tonifies the liver and the flow of Ch'i in the liver.

This was followed by giving pressure over Li-4 as shown in the figure, this point is known by the name 'adjoining valley' and is known to be the master point in removing stagnation in the flow of Ch'i thereby making the rest of the treatment much easier and more effective. Pressure over this point should not be given to the pregnant women. Thereafter pressed St-36, in conjunction with Sp-6. Whereas giving pressure over St-36 helps in alleviating tired muscles and general fatigue, it is known to strengthen the whole body, aids digestion, and relieves stomach disorders by stimulating intestinal functioning. Giving pressure over Sp-6, the 'three Yin meeting point' located above the ankle bone towards the inside of the leg on the back side, is known to be one of the best points since it strengthens three meridians, viz. kidneys, liver and spleen at the same time and helps flush the Ch'i and blood through the body. Thereafter, I gave pressure over Cv-6 and Cv-12 points. Whereas Cv-6, known as "sea of energy" is located three finger widths below the naval and is known to relieve abdominal pain, colitis and gas formation, Cv-12, as its name 'middle stomach' itself suggests is located midway between the breast bone and the belly button. The famous combination of Cv-6; Cv-12 and St-25 which is known as 'four doors' is highly beneficial to overcome any type of stomach or gastrointestinal disorders. This was followed by giving pressure over St-25, which is located two thumb widths from the vertebral column on both sides, at the back of belly button. Pressure over this point has to be given on both sides simultaneously with medium yet firm pressure for 30 seconds to one minute to get best results. At the end gave pressure over Sp-4 which is known by the name 'grandfather-grandson' point. To locate this point, commence from the joint where the big toe connects to the foot. Slide along the bone and from the middle of the joint move three finger widths towards the ankle. Sp-4 is just there as shown in the figure.

Surprisingly, the patient responded beyond expectations, and the very third day when I went to him for giving him the therapy, I was informed by the mother of my friend that your patient has been asking for food since yesterday night but she had not given her much beyond what was allowed. She reported, he has been going round the home where as he had been lying in the bed for past many days. I gave him the therapy and came back after allowing him dalia/rice cooked thoroughly with moong dal in semi-solid form. Next day when I went for giving the therapy and asked what his Homeopathic physician told him and asked him to take the medicine given to him by the Homeopath meticulously, to my utter surprise, I was informed they had cancelled the appointment in view of the substantial improvement he had made within three sessions of acupressure. After giving seven sessions to him daily (once), I told him that now we can go for the sessions every alternate day. He resumed his duties. Looking into his recovery, the patient and my friend insisted that now they can come to my home so that I save my time on transit. In all the treatment lasted for three weeks more, i.e. in all about 15-16 sessions and the patient had recovered completely.

□

Case–8
Sciatica/Insomnia

I recall the case of Mr. B, a retired DIG from para-military forces, who was brought to me, in the year 1999, with severe shooting pain in his left leg that was diagnosed to be due to 'sciatica', as also insomnia partly because of the excruciating pain and otherwise too the patient had been very often on sleeping pills, as reported to me. The intensity of the pain was so high that his wife and son who had accompanied him told me that every day he is on heavy dose of pain killers of the sort of 'Tremadol-50 mg', at times thrice a day. In the night they used to give him two capsules of Tremadol-50 mg, one tablet each of Combiflam and 0.5 mg of Alprex, and tie crape bandage on his leg in their bid to give him relief, but despite all these measures, he was not able to sleep due to the excruciating pain he had and used to cry at the top of his voice, disturbing even the neighbors. He had been referred to me by one of my patients who had successfully undergone treatment from Acupressure therapy, for his Cervical Spondylosis some time back, at my clinic.

Although, prior to this, I had handled many patients suffering from sciatica pain yet perhaps this was the most critical case I had come across. In a majority of cases, the problem is accompanied by severe pain radiating from hip joint towards the ankle joint, at times even to the extent that the pain radiates to the entire leg accompanied with excruciating pain so much so that the patient finds it difficult

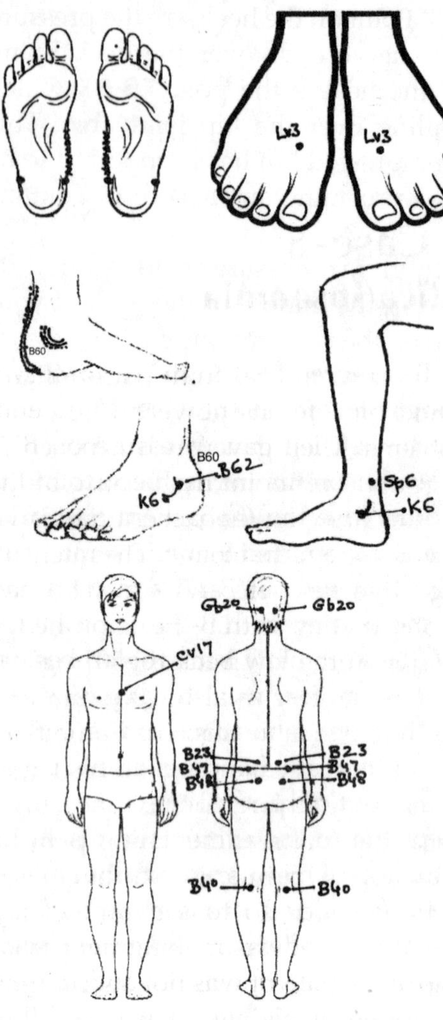

to even move his leg/foot. Most of the times this problem has stress; improper posture, injury or weak muscles as the underlying cause at its back, however in the instant case no injury as such had been reported. The treatment commenced with stimulating the entire left sole. With a view to provide a bit of immediate relief, I gave pressure over the entire sole using 'thumb walk' technique for about 2-3 minutes, followed by giving massage like pressure over the Achilles tendon area (the area behind the leg above the heel). This is the area from where the sciatic nerve passes behind the ankles and goes down to the bottom of the heels, on both anterior and posterior sides of the heel. This was followed by giving pressure over the 'lumbo-sacral' area of the vertebral column, marked as 'xxxxxx' and other points in the figure. This was done keeping in mind the fact that often sciatica pain is also caused by the nerve compression or a slip-disc in the lumbosaccral area. Point on the heels are the pressure points where the sciatic nerve ends over the heel. Point, shown on the back of the heel is the point 'B-60' which pertains to the area falling over the hip joint area. This point hurts a lot on being pressed but has been found to be extremely beneficial in overcoming any sort of discomfort in the lower back area.

This was followed by giving pressure over B-40 (middle of the crooke), is located in the middle of the back of your knee, in the centre between the two tendons over the crease formed when you bend your knee. This point is also known by the name 'Command Point' for its powerful influence on the lower back problems. Then gave pressure on B-23 point, as shown in the figure. This point has been found to be of immense help in alleviating lower back pain, sciatica and fatigue caused due to severe pain in that area. This was followed by giving pressure over B-47, as shown, this point when pressed in conjunction with B-23, helps a lot in providing relief in the pain in the low back region besides helping in overcoming fatigue, fear as also calming down the irritated sciatic nerve. Further to this, I pressed B-48, which helps provide relief in sciatica, hip pain, lower back pain and in alleviating tension in the region.

Coming to the other aspect of his ailment, i.e. insomnia, which in the instant case, was primarily attributable to uneven distribution of energy or so to say non-smooth transition from Yang to Yin cycle, was making the patient irritable and restless. Since the patient was not able to sleep for at least 6-7 hrs., required at his age, it was resulting into overloading of certain meridians while blocking of certain others. To overcome the situation, started with giving pressure over Lv-3. This point helps in neutralizing all types of stress and has a calming/relaxing effect on the mind. Pressed Sp-6, three Yin meeting point, to help flush Ch'i and blood through the body. The combination of the Yin nourishing and calming effect makes it instrumental in getting rid of insomnia. Next point to be pressed was Gb-20 which is located in the hollow below the base of the skull. Mild to moderate pressure should be given on this point on both sides, and as its name suggests, i.e. 'gates of consciousness' , this point is known to overcome stiffness in the region of the neck besides eliminating the effect of wind and cold and overcoming the problem of insomnia. Also gave pressure over Cv-17, known as Sea of Tranquility, on the centre of the breast bone, it relieves anxiety, has calming effect over the nerves and thereby helps in overcoming insomnia.

This was followed by giving pressure over B-62, 'Calm Sleep', found on the outer side of the ankle in the indentation. It helps relieve back pain that makes it difficult for the patient to sleep. To end the session, pressure was given on K-6, 'Joyful Sleep' point, which is found in the indentation below the inner side of the ankle, to relieve anxiety and get rid of insomnia. Finally, I gave pressure over the reflex point pertaining to the Pineal gland, which is known to control the sleep pattern in our body with a view to overcome the problem of sleeplessness in the patient, the area to be pressed has been shown in figure, gave pressure for about 30-40 seconds over this point in all the four limbs.

By the time the treatment was over, which took nearly 45 mins., it was around 8.30 pm. Normally, I ask the therapy to be repeated after around 18-24 hours, but in the instant case looking into the intensity/severity of the pain, I asked the son of the patient to bring him again for the therapy the next day around 10 am, being Sunday. I also advised him not to take so many pain killers at a time since that may lead to other major problems and advised him to take minimum amount of pain killers. Next day when the patient came, I asked him how he spent his night and how many pain killers he had to take? Before his son or wife could say any thing, he asked them to keep quite and said I want to narrate. He lifted both his hands in the air, thanking God and uttered "Aaraaam raha…ek bhi pain killer nahi liya… bandage bhi nahi bandhi…sab ko aaraam se sone diya…aur khud bhi chain se soya!!!

Frankly speaking, I myself was not prepared for this sort of a response so soon. That is what I want to convey through this case is that it all depends upon the body response and no doubt to some extent on the faith of the patient. Whereas, the instant case cannot be quoted as a case for body response for one and all, yet in a major number of cases you will find that relief in the intensity of pain is instant, provided the pressure is given the right way, at the right point, to the right extent and for the right duration. That is why I say, in case you do not get relief, blame the therapist not the therapy, for the therapy is fool proof. His treatment lasted for about 12 sessions.

□

Case–9
Paralysis/Loss of Voice

About six months back, a student of mine phoned me that her maternal uncle, aged around 62 years has suffered a paralytic stroke, has a total loss of voice and is not able to lift his right limbs. He had come from a place called Saifai in Uttar Pradesh and was hospitalized in a hospital of repute in Greater Noida. I told her to attend her uncle herself as and when she visits him in the hospital and asked her to come along with the son of the patient, so that they could be briefed as to how to go about the treatment. But she was not confident as she had taken training only a few months back. When they came, I asked her in case she remembered the points to be pressed and I was happy to note that she remembered most of the pressure points required to be pressed in the instant case. But they informed that the patient has been in the hospital for almost 12 days with no sign of recovery and they intended to bring him home in Noida. They insisted that I should visit the patient at least once. On visiting the patient, I found that the family members were not very much enthusiastic in handling the case by themselves, despite the fact that I was willing to spend some time to train 2-3 of them. My student while taking me to their home, on the way expressed her inability to go there every day, as distance from her home was around 33 kms one way. Finally, I had to agree to attend the patient. I advised them to continue with the treatment that was being given in the hospital, as also to keep in constant

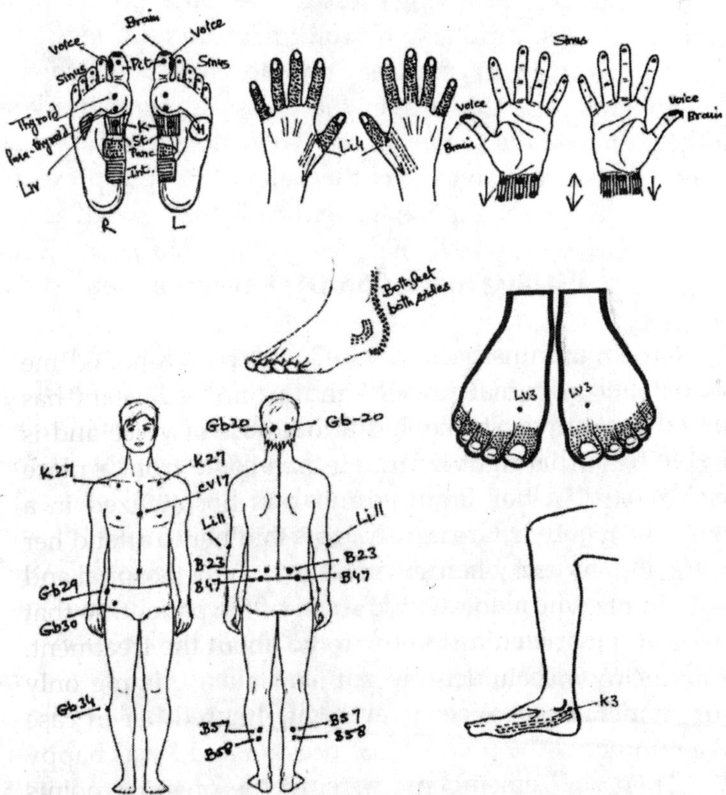

touch with the attending physician while continuing to take acupressure treatment. In other words, we resorted to co-management.

As I had guessed, discussions revealed that the patient had been suffering from hypertension and he did not take any medicine for 2-3 days due to some function in the family and one night he suffered the stroke, the most common manifestation of stroke due to cerebral hemorrhage resulting from hypertension. To begin with, I started giving pressure over the point marked in figure (on both soles). This pressure point pertains to the brain. Since right side of the body had been effected, more emphasis had to be given on the left foot and palm so far as this point is concerned.

This was followed by giving pressure over other point which refer to sinuses, pituitary, thyroid, para-thyroid, kidneys, stomach, liver, heart, pancreas and adrenals respectively. Pressure was also given over the pressure points marked in the palms on the same pattern. Thereafter, pressure was given both on the soles and the palms over the pressure point marked in the inner edge of the big toes as well as the thumbs. Giving pressure over these points has been found to be very effective for the purpose of restoration of the lost voice.

Next point pressed was Gb-20 which is known by the name 'gates of consciousness' and is located in the hollow below the base of the skull, and has been considered to be highly beneficial in overcoming the stiffness in the region of the neck as well as in eliminating the wind and cold present, thereby restoring the energy imbalance(s), if any in the kidney and bladder meridians. Also press B-23 and B-47 points whose location is shown in figure, these points are useful in providing relief in the lower back region and in reducing muscle tension, fatigue trauma, etc., gave firm but moderate pressure over each point for 30 seconds to a minute.

Thereafter, applied pressure over K-27 and K-3 points, as shown. They are known to stimulate the 'Yin' and sedate the 'Yang' of liver and kidneys. For maximum benefit ask the patient to inhale and exhale breath deeply. Also gave pressure over Li-4 (Adjoining Valley) and Li-11 (Crooked Pond). Whereas Li-4 eliminates the toxins through the bowels, it is helpful in overcoming stagnation in Ch'i too. Li-11 helps restore energy flow thereby benefiting the large intestines and the lung meridians. Followed by this, I pressed Cv-17, this point is known by the name 'Sea of tranquility', this lies on the centre of the breast bone as shown, and considered to be one of the best points for balancing the small intestines and the heart meridian and is extremely useful in establishing 'emotional' balance in our body. Pressing Lv-3, a point which has been found to be most essential pressure point and can be pressed for help in almost any ailment connected to either of the systems in our body. It regulates and tonifies the liver meridian and the 'Ch'i in the liver meridian besides overcoming the damage caused to the gallbladder and liver meridians, besides detoxification.

Follow this by giving pressure over Gb-34, known by the name 'Sunny side of the Mountain', this point lies in the depression below the bony prominence on the lateral side of the knee. This points dispels wind, clears damp heat and stimulates the liver's 'Yin'. Liver nourishes the joints, mobility of the joint, muscular strain is improved by giving pressure over this point. Gb-30 known as "Jumping Circle", and Gb-29 are other important points, as shown in the figure, are very useful for relieving hip joint problem besides stimulating circulation in the entire leg and low back. Since the muscle in this part of the body is sufficiently thicker, in case you are not able to reach this point with the help of your thumbs (one over the other — to exert double pressure), pressure can be given with the help of your elbow, but very cautiously. Also press B-57 (Support the Mountain) and B-58, as shown in figure, to get relief in leg pain and also stiffness in that area.

It has been noticed that once the recovery process sets in, first of all the lost voice is regained. Thereafter, the patient regains the movement of the legs, i.e. the patient starts raising his effected leg(s), bending it and last of all the upper limb(s) (which generally take a lot of time) start responding. At this stage in case help of a physiotherapist is also taken, the recovery process is further accelerated.

Giving pressure over the upper part of the big toes, thumbs and the fingers of both the feet and the hands (the portion shown with the help of shade, i.e. dots as shown is the figure has been found to be highly beneficial to stimulate the neuro system. This can be done with ease with the help of a Spring Ring which is easily available in the market, in the absence of which pressure on these areas can be given with the help of a comb or a hair brush or with the help of the tip of a match stick. Under no circumstances this area should be neglected. This should be followed by giving pressure around the ankles and behind the heel on the area shown with the help of dotted lines (Achilles tendons) as also the area shown with the help of dotted lines commencing from the joint of the big toe leading towards the heel (see figure). Pressure should also be given over the channels 1 to 4 as marked over both the feet and the upper part of the hands (see figure). Last of all pressure may also be given over the shaded portion of the wrists, points to, this area stimulates the genitals and thus helps in strengthening the muscles of the lower back. As has been stated earlier too, for the first 3-4 sessions all the aforesaid pressure points needs to be touched upon every day, thereafter, some of the pressure points may be omitted on one day and may be touched upon the other day and vice versa.

Another point that needs a special mention here is that recovery amongst the patients suffering from this sort of ailments depends to a great extent on the willpower of the patient to get well soon, for the reason that until and unless the patient tries to move his limbs himself, which he is not able to move because of the ailment, they would become further stiff. That is why, it is said that 50% of the recovery in such cases comes from the willpower of the patient and rest of the recovery is attained from treatment/medication. Body weight of the patient is yet another important factor. Patients with relatively less weight get well sooner than the obese patients. In the instant case, unfortunately this patient had to be forced to try to move his limbs and did not exhibit much initiative on his own, despite that, whereas he regained his voice by the time we reached 8th session, further recovery took around 25 sessions for the patient to become able to move by holding the chair. The treatment could not continue as the patient insisted to go back home and almost forced his people to take him back to his home town. As such the people around him had to be taught as to how and where to give pressure. I was given to understand by my student that his wife and nephew insisted and continued to give him pressure and now he has recovered so much that he moves out of his home, even alone, though with the support of a walker.

□

Case–10
Neuralgia; Cervical

In the year 1991, one of my patients came to me and asked that in case 'acupressure' therapy could be of any help in handling a patient suffering from 'Neuralgia' and Cervical Spondylosis. He said one of his seniors in office, an IAS officer had been suffering from Cervical problem for more than 3-4 years and for about an year or so the problem has further aggravated since 'Neuralgasic' pain has developed. I told him whereas Cervical part can be handled with much ease, about the Neuralgia part, there was no harm in making an effort. The appointment was fixed for the week end. During the course of the discussions with the patient, it was learnt that his Cervical problem was pretty old may be 7-8 years and that he had learnt to live with it, but the Neuralgic pain was troubling him a lot. He informed me that many a time while shaving, when he reaches a particular spot near his chin, he feels as if he has got an electric shock and many a time he gets a cut over his skin. I could guess that his Trigeminal Nerve might have become too irritated and the moment the razor touches it he gets shock like sensation. As a matter of fact, Neuralgia, is a sort of nerve pain occurring when the nerve is irritated or inflamed. The pain spreading along neural pathways may be acute or chronic and may range from mild to unbearable. When the multi-branched cranial nerve is effected neuralgia accompanied with facial pain is termed 'Trigeminal Neuralgia'. This problem occurs generally in people of the age group of 50 and above, women

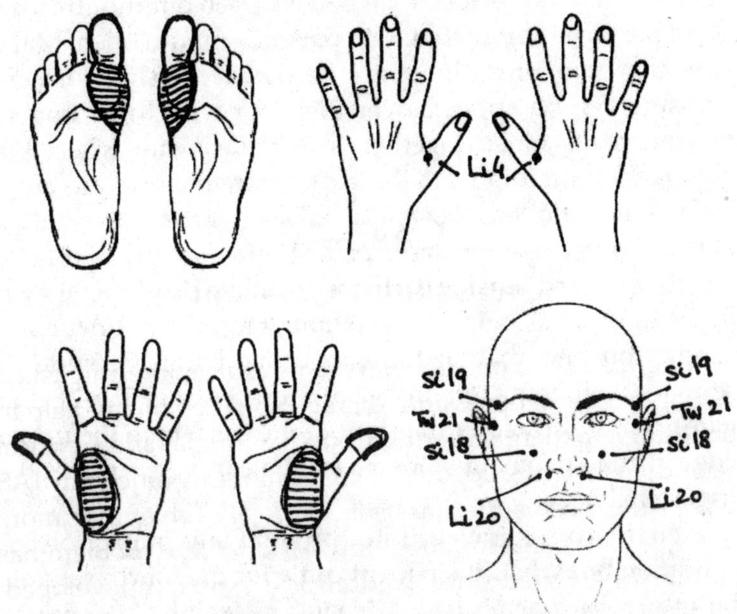

are more prone to this ailment. The type of pain may be sudden, shooting, sharp, burning or stabbing, itching or aching. Generally on one side, may be intermittent or at time continuous. May last for days or at times for weeks. The pain at times becomes unbearable.

I commenced his treatment, stimulating the reflex areas around both of his big toes and the thumbs, followed by giving rolling pressure over the pads below the big toes in the soles and the same below the thumbs. Over Li-4, the 'adjoining valley', which is considered to be one of the most effective points to treat infections in ENT area as well as by its pain killing effect too. Pregnant women should not press this point. This was followed by giving pressure over Si-18, a point known as 'Cheek Bone Hole', that lies below the outside edge of the eye in an indentation below the zygomatic bone. It relieves pain over the face, helpful in overcoming facial paralysis and trigeminal neuralgia. Next point to be pressed was Si-19, this point lies in the depression which is formed when we open our mouth. This point has to be stimulated with patient's mouth open. Make sure that you press in centre of the depression formed, pressure can be applied over this area with three fingers of your hand joined together. This is the point where the gallbladder meridian and the triple warmer meridians cross each other and has beneficial effect over the trigeminal nerve to overcome the nerve pain. Thereafter, pressed Li-20 which is located outside each nostril on the cheeks as shown in the figure, this helps in overcoming facial swelling, nasal congestion and that in the sinuses and thus provides a sense of well-being. Finally gave pressure over Tw-21 (Ear gate), that is located at the front of the ear where the upper edge of the zygomatic bone meets the ear. It stimulates the trigeminal nerve.

First two sessions did not provide any impact on his condition but when the patient came for the fourth session, he informed that he had a feeling of well-being, though the pain recurred but the intensity was less severe. This inculcated some faith in the patient in the therapy, since despite taking injections of alcohol over the effected nerve, he could never get that feeling of well-being, that he was having now, although he reported that the pain used to subside for some days after each shot. After 7th session, I asked him to take treatment every alternate day and in all I gave him 15 sessions for a long-term recovery. Over these years since then, he had only two relapses and on each occasion, he approached me immediately and got relief in barely 4-5 sessions. Since then he has been recommending patients suffering from ailments of varied nature confidently. He even wrote a letter of appreciation to me acknowledging his gratitude and recommending expansion of this sort of therapies which have great healing potential.

□

Case–11
Heel Pain

Mr. A, a senior bureaucrat from Civil Services, consulted me for his heel pain, somewhere in the year 1998. He was a keen player of lawn tennis, but due to his heel pain, he was not able to play. Even in his day-to-day conduct, his heel pain was proving to be a great impediment. This sort of pain is most common in the players, pain is worst while rising up from the bed in the morning, bearing weight over the heel after one gets up after sitting for a long time. Stiffness & intensity of the pain reduces with activity. However, the pain returns after prolonged activity. Maximum pain is felt on the medial aspect of the calcanium. In some of the cases, it is seen that obesity may be the underlying cause and whereas in other cases, some problem with the genitals too has also been found to be one of the causative factors behind such a problem.

Pressure was given around the arch of the foot, as shown by 'xxxxx' area marked in figure, with a view to stimulate the lumbo sacral part of the vertebral column, for about a minute on each side. This was followed by giving pressure as shown in figure, the shaded area over the wrist of both hands on both sides by giving pressure in the direction indicated with the help of an arrow, after having stimulated this area for about a minute or so, give pressure over points marked in the figure. Thereafter gave pressure around the ankles of both the feet, in particular over the effected feet, down the dotted lines as shown in figure. Pressure was also

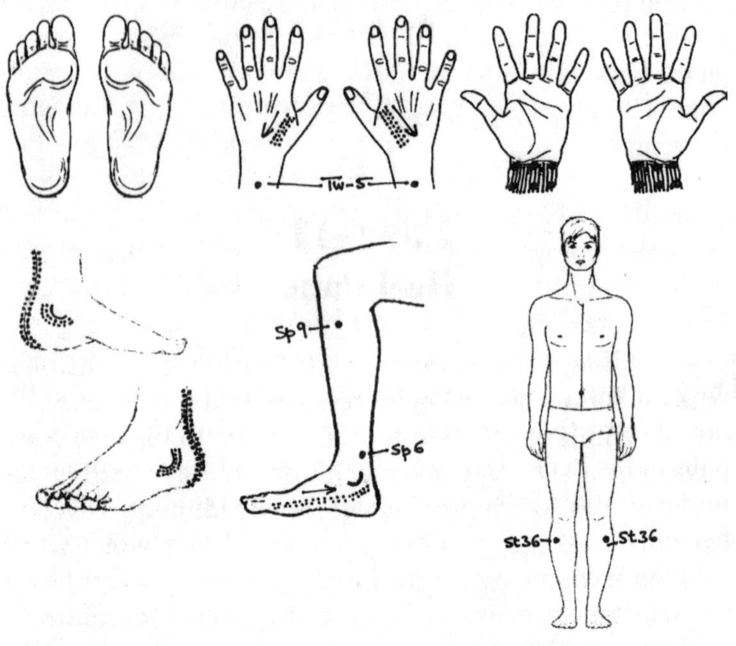

given over Achilles tendon area shown with the help of dotted lines. Also gave pressure over the area depicted by the dotted lines in the figures over the back of the palms and the anterior side of the feet, in the indicated direction. It has been observed that giving pressure over these areas which has a direct impact over the nervous system, provides much relief to the patients suffering from heel pain. This was followed by giving pressure over Tw-5 point (at times massage-like pressure has to be given over this point as it gets tender very soon), this point lies on the back of the wrist, about three finger widths from the wrist crease, as shown in the figure. Giving pressure over this point has also been found to be extremely beneficial in over coming heel pain. Further to this, gave pressure over St-36, which lies four finger widths below the knee cap, one thumb width on the outside of the shin bone. This point strengthens the entire body, tones the muscles particularly when given in combination with Sp-6 (Three Yin Meeting Point) which is located above the ankle bone towards the inside of the leg on the back side — about four finger widths above the ankle bone. This point is considered as the most potent point since it strengthens the Yin of three meridians simultaneously. It is also considered to be best pressure point to overcome any gynecological problem, if any. Pregnant women should not press this point. Also pressed Sp-9 which lies on the inside of the leg, under the shin bone and is known to overcome any sort of edema in the lower part of the body.

The treatment lasted for around 12 sessions and Mr. A wrote a letter to me informing about the recovery and that now he can play three sets in a row without getting any pain in his heels. His wife, who is also a senior bureaucrat underwent a crash course and could later on help her father herself who had suffered an 'Angina attack' soon after her training was over.

□

Case–12
Slip Disc/Sciatica

Some time in the year 2003, Mr. G, a retired top ranking officer from Rajasthan aged about 68 years, was admitted to a renowned hospital of New Delhi with Prolapsed Disc problem under the care of an orthopedic surgeon of international repute and was advised surgery. Immediate surgery could not be performed because of some other complications which needed to be taken care of in the first instance. Another senior officer from the same state who was also holding a senior position and had some exposure to the efficacy of acupressure therapy, suggested to him to have acupressure therapy along with the treatment he was having, while waiting for the surgery to get at least some relief from the severe pain he was suffering, to which he agreed. Since I was slated to visit the States after about 11 days, we decided to give him two sessions per day, one in the morning and another in the evening for the first few days, looking into the severity of the pain and time available at our disposal.

Since his son-in-law who was also a medico, was accompanying him, there was not much of a problem in making the patient understand, the underlying cause. I started with giving a thumb walk over both the soles for about 2-3 minutes each sole, to provide him some relief, though superficially in the beginning. This was followed by giving rolling pressure over the Lumbo sacral area, i.e in the arch of the foot. Thereafter, I gave pressure on specific points

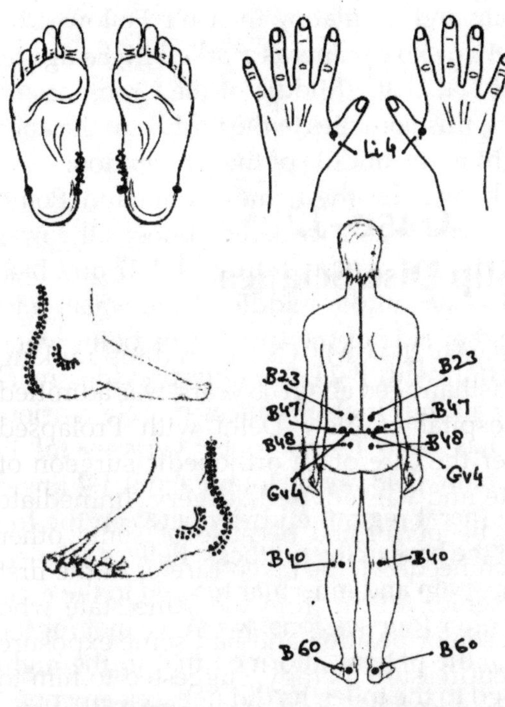

pertaining to L4-L5 and S-1-2, since this was the area where the disc had been herniated. Thereafter I gave pressure over the points as shown in the figure. Pressure over these points was given to stimulate the sciatic nerve endings.

Sciatic nerve ends in the base of the sole at these points and it has been seen that in most of the cases of disc prolapse/slip disc, sciatic nerve is irritated because of the compression over the sciatic nerve which is caused by the rupture of the disc.

Pressure has also to be given over the points marked, i.e. around the ankles and the Achilles tendon area depicted by the shaded portion (dotted lines) and the point shown about 1-1/4′ from the base of the heel, this pertains to the sacral region, is very sensitive to touch but is highly beneficial in over coming any sort of pain in the lower back area. Then give pressure over B-60, as shown in the figure. It relieves back pain in the lower and upper back as also the legs. This may be followed by giving pressure over Gv-4, which can be located at the waistline about 2-3 finger widths below the B-23 point, to get relief from pain. Pressure has also to be given over Li-4, adjoining valley, which is known for its ability to relieve pain and circulating the Ch'i. Followed by giving pressure on two extra points as marked in the figure. Next point pressed was B-40, 'Middle of the Crook', as its name itself suggests, this point lies in the middle of the knee when it is bent, right in the middle of the two tendons.

This point is known by the name 'Command Point' because of its powerful influence over almost all lower back problems. To end the session, I pressed B-47 and B-48 points. Whereas B-47 lies in the middle of the waist, four finger widths on either side of the spine. This point when pressed in conjunction with B-23, not only provides relief in the lower back pain but it also reduces muscle tension, fatigue, fear and has been found to be very useful in alleviating sciatica pain, B-48 can be found about 1-2 finger widths outside the sacral region, midway between the top of the hip bone and the base of the buttocks. Relives sciatica, hip pain, lower back pain and muscular tension in the area.

Third day, i.e. after four sessions, when we met for the fifth session, Mr. G, the patient informed that in the night when he got up to go to the toilet, he did not seek any ones' help and could make it to the toilet on his own, though slowly. As such we decided that after giving two more sessions the same day, we shall meet only once in a day thereafter. In all, before the date of my departure, 13 sittings were given and the patient was in a fairly good condition, stopped taking any pain killers. When I came back and enquired about the welfare of Mr. G, from the officer who had recommended him for the treatment, I was informed that when he went for consultation with the surgeon, as scheduled, after check up the patient was told that surgery was no more required.

□

Case–13
Prostate

Mr. B, a senior IPS officer, aged about 54 years, was recommended for treatment at my clinic by one of his colleagues in the year 2003, for his prostate problem. He informed me that he had been suffering from this problem for almost more than 4-5 years, but of late the problem has become so acute that at times he finds it extremely inconvenient to handle., He informed that he has to get up to urinate three to four times during the night and it takes quite some time in voiding the bladder or to hold the urine during the meetings, in case the meeting gets prolonged. He further informed that even after passing the urine, a few drops dribble out, again a difficult and embarrassing situation.

Prostate is an ailment which most of the males suffer at one time or the other in their life, any time after the age of 45 or so. As a matter of fact, prostate is a gland located midway between the scrotum and anus, below bladder in the males. It produces and secretes fluids that accompany the sperm, protecting it on its way to the Cervix. It surrounds the Urethra, the tube that carries urine from the bladder through the penis. Enlarged prostate restricts the smooth flow of urine through the urethra and as a result thereof they have to get up for urination in the night as reported in this case. Other accompanying conditions could be slow urination, difficult to commence, dribbling after passing urine and at times the patient has burning sensation during or after urination.

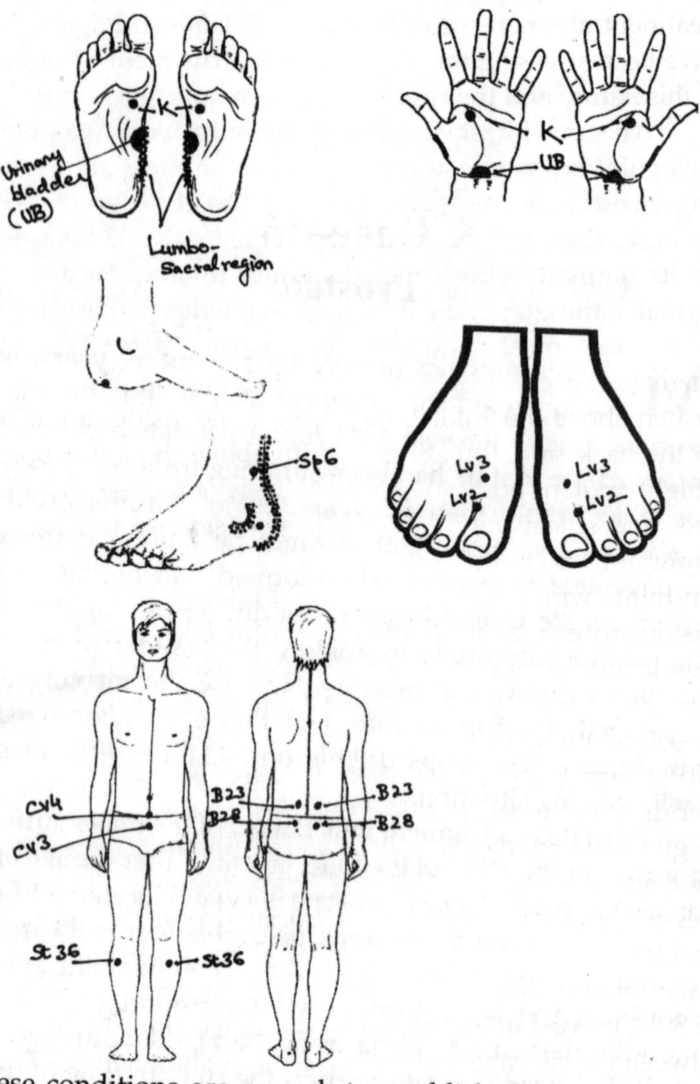

These conditions are enough to establish the onset of the disease which is generally confined to inflammation of the prostate. It would be wise to get yourself examined by your family physician, in case you feel that you have even some of the afore-said symptoms, with a view to rule out the probability of malignancy, before going in for any sort of treatment, the non-conventional way. Time and again, we have been stressing the need for co-management of case(s) of this nature and the results have been quite encouraging.

To begin with, started giving pressure over LV-3 point. This point lies between the big and second toe, about two finger width above Lv-2 point which lies at the junction of the big and second toe, on the top of the foot. Lv-3 is known for its tonifying effect over the entire immune system. It regulated the Ch'i in the liver meridian which is considered to be the most powerful organ for 'detoxification'. Thereafter, pressed Sp-6, the three meeting point, which is located above the ankle bone towards the inside of the leg on the back side, four finger width above the ankle bone, a highly potent point to simultaneously stimulate kidneys, liver and spleen meridians and is considered to be very important for providing relief in the instant condition. In continuity with this point pressure should be given at St. 36, this pressure point strengthens the entire body, tones up the muscles and revitalizes the entire body. Next point pressed was Cv-3, which is located about one thumb width below Cv-4 (known as Gate Origin) which is located four finger widths below the belly button. Its effect over the 'bladder meridian' is almost specific. Pressure over this point should be given after emptying the bladder. Stimulate this point for a few minutes, gently. This can be followed by giving pressure at B-28, which is an associated point for urinary bladder, located at about one and a half inches on either side of the spine as shown in the figure. Thereafter give pressure on B-23, located in the middle of the waist, almost half way between the rib cage and the hip bone as shown in fig. This point is known for its effect on sexual reproductivity organs and as a result helps in over coming prostate problem. Giving final touches to the session, gave pressure around the ankles of both the feet on both anterior and posterior sides as shown by the dotted lines in the figure as also over the mid point between the lowest portion of the ankle and the heel (diagonally) as shown in the figure. Followed by giving rolling pressure over the reflex area relating to the urinary bladder which lies in the lumbo sacral part of the spine with a view to strengthen the urinary bladder.

After just two sessions, Mr. B reported some relief and informed that instead of getting up four times the previous night, he had to get up only two times and the time taken in emptying the bladder was also comparatively much less, the burning sensation had almost gone, but dribbling was still there. In all 11 sessions proved to be sufficient to bring substantial relief.

□

Case–14
Arthritis (Rheumatoid)

A relation of mine who had been a professor in JNU one day called me to discuss the case of one of his colleagues in the same university whose wife, 52 years, had been suffering from severe arthritis. He informed me that the patient was in such a bad state that she was bed ridden for more than three months and that I will have to visit them. On one of the weekends, we decided to visit them. I was taken to their residence and the professor whose wife was ailing had to drag her to the sitting room in a chair as she was not able to get up/move.

The patient was really in a very bad state, there was almost no movement in her pelvic joints, she was not able to even open her palms, over all it was a bad case of rheumatoid arthritis. On the top of it, their house was far away from my residence and commuting there every day was a real problem. The professor told me that he will arrange for my pick up and dropping and we agreed that for a week I will attend her every day and during this period I shall try to train the professor to administer the therapy himself. I told him very clearly the first day itself that it is any body's guess as to how effective the therapy would be, when introduced at such a late stage. Much damage had already been done. He had exhausted probably all channels of treatment without success and lastly he thought of trying out acupressure therapy too, hoping against hope!!

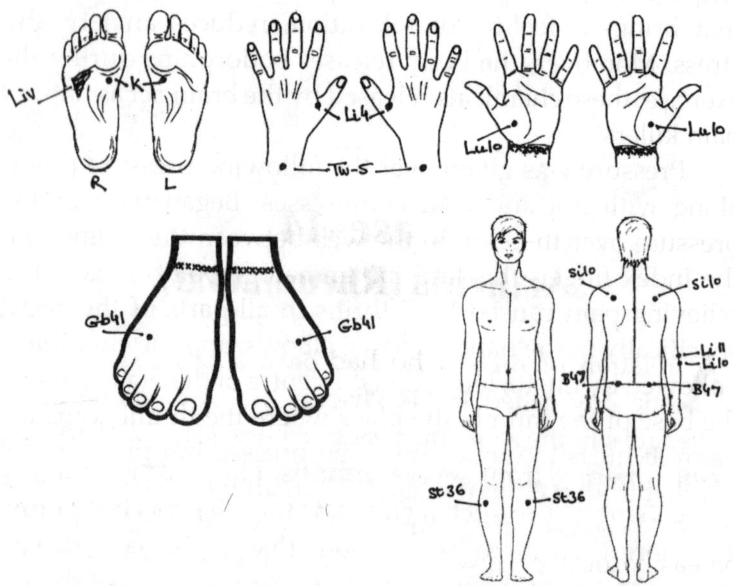

Many types of arthritis are known, yet most of them may be grouped into two categories, viz. (a) Osteoarthritis (OA) and Rheumatoid Arthritis (RA). The word 'Arthritis' means inflammation of the joints. This case was a confirmation of the findings of a study published in July 2002 in the journal *Arthritis and Rheumatism*, which read "if you do not move around and keep your muscles and joints flexible, your arthritic symptoms will worsen". They had concluded that those who avoided activity during a painful arthritic flare up, were more prone to be disabled as compared to the people who continued activity, though with some amount of modifications. In another study, researchers had found that the women with rheumatoid arthritis, who had the thickest thigh muscles also had denser femur bone. This finding supports the importance of movement and exercise for keeping the muscle strong and bone mobile and strong for preventing the fractures caused by osteoporosis. Exercise may also be the most effective treatment as it helps to relieve deep muscle pain, fatigue, and other symptoms.

Regular exercise produces 'Alpha waves' in the brain that brings a feeling of relaxation, reduces anxiety and stress. Moreover, the body releases endorphins during the exercise; these chemicals released by the brain act as natural pain killers.

Pressure was given over the following pressure points along with hot and cold compresses: Began with giving pressure over the Li-4, in the web between the thumb and the index finger, this anti-inflammatory point is useful in relieving pain caused by arthritis in all parts of the body, specifically in the hands, wrists, elbows, and the shoulders. Followed by Lu-10, located in the centre of the big mound at the base of the thumb, the place where the thumb joins the palm. It hurts too much on being pressed but provides lot of relief from pain in the hand. Thereafter look for the Tw-5 point. In case you flex your hand backwards, this point can be easily located between Ulna and Radius bones around three finger widths from the wrist crease. Press firmly. This points removes stress from the shoulders as well as helps in getting relief from pain in the entire arm, besides toning up the muscles. Next point pressed was Li-10, just below the Li-11 point which is found over the end of the crease that is formed when you bend you hand and try to hold your shoulder. This point is also considered to be an anti-inflammatory point that helps relieve arthritic discomfort in the hands, wrists, and the elbow joints besides giving relief to aching muscles and joints due to arthritis. Arthritic patients should be taught to make it a habit to stimulate this point on both the arms when they get up in the morning. Point Li-11 should be pressed very softly with modest pressure, as this point, though of great importance, gets very tender to touch, as such needs to be stimulated with great care. It relieves inflammation of the elbow and shoulder joints. Also an important point to overcome allergies of various kinds.

Followed by pressing Si-10, as shown in the figure. Press on the muscular cord of the shoulder joint, is known to relieve arthritis, bursitis, and rheumatism. Relieves shoulder and upper back pain. After having given pressure as stated above press B-47, which is located on the lower back between second and third Lumber vertebrae about 1-1/2" away from spine on its either sides. It relieves lower backache and fatigue. Next point pressed was St-36, about four finger widths below the knee cap and one thumb width outside the shin bone. Helps in overcoming arthritic pain all over the body and in particular the pain in the knee joints, is considered to be the most potent pressure points for alleviating sore, tired muscles, and fatigue. Strengthens the whole body, tones up the muscles. Also pressed Gb-41, can be located (about two finger widths from the joint between the little and second finger) above the fourth and fifth metatarsal bones. This point, besides overcoming knee pain, has been found to be of immense use in overcoming hip and shoulder tension, rheumatism, excessive water retention and in reducing stress over sciatic nerve. With a view to provide relief to the pelvic joint, pressure was given in the lymphatic area as well, i.e. where the feet and the leg join together, as also at the joint where the palm and the lower hand meet, i.e. wrist crease. Both these areas have been found to be of immense use in over coming any problem/pain in the groin area. The areas to be stimulated has been shown by "xxxxxxxxx" in the figure.

In case treatment is commenced at the onset of the disease itself, the patient can be saved to a great extent from arthritic changes that take place in the shape of deformity. However, as in the instant case when treatment was started at a very late stage, where as nothing can be done towards restoring the deformity, but further damage can be checked to a great extent. A lot still depends on the body response of each individual. The instant case was reported so late that up to 5-6 sessions, no relief worth making a mention was noticed except that the patient reported that the extent of discomfort and intensity of pain has somewhat reduced.

The female started responding after around eight sessions to the extent that she could turn in the bed herself, though still with some discomfort, I was asked to continue treatment for yet another week. Looking into some improvement in the overall condition of the patient, I agreed and by the time 14 sessions were given without any break, she had started sitting on her own in her bed. By this time her husband had learnt to give therapy and he took over on the condition that every Sunday, I will be coming to attend her. The total treatment lasted for about four months, her husband also took lot of interest and started doing it too well with practice and once she started moving in side her house with the help of a walker, I stopped going to attend the patient. It took almost an year before she could climb down the stairs of her home at the first floor and come to my clinic to thank me. □

Case–15
Piles (Hemorrhoids)

An old patient of mine, who had taken treatment of water retention some years back contacted me to find out in case 'acupressure therapy' could be of some help in getting rid of 'Piles'? I told her that in 'acupressure therapy' we do not go on the basis of disease, but we go by the 'holistic approach', i.e. we treat the body as a whole and not the disease specifically. Told her that we try to remove the root cause of the disease and once the cause is removed, the problem to which we give the name of a disease automatically disappears. On asking who the patient was, she informed that her mother who was in Himachal Pradesh has been having harrowing time with the piles problem and that she has been suffering from this problem for more than 10 years or so. Having bleeding and painful piles. She said that since she has been advised surgery, she was planning to get her to Delhi in a day or two. I told her to bring the patient to me and give me four to five days time before taking a final decision for going in for surgery, to which she agreed.

Here, let me make it clear as to why I sought 4-5 days time? This was for the reason that over the years of my practice healing patients coming from all walks of life with problems of varied nature, I have observed that by and large, barring the cases of extremely chronic nature, in case the body response of the patient is fine, the patient, within three or at best four sessions starts feeling the change(s) within his/her body. Going by that experience, generally I

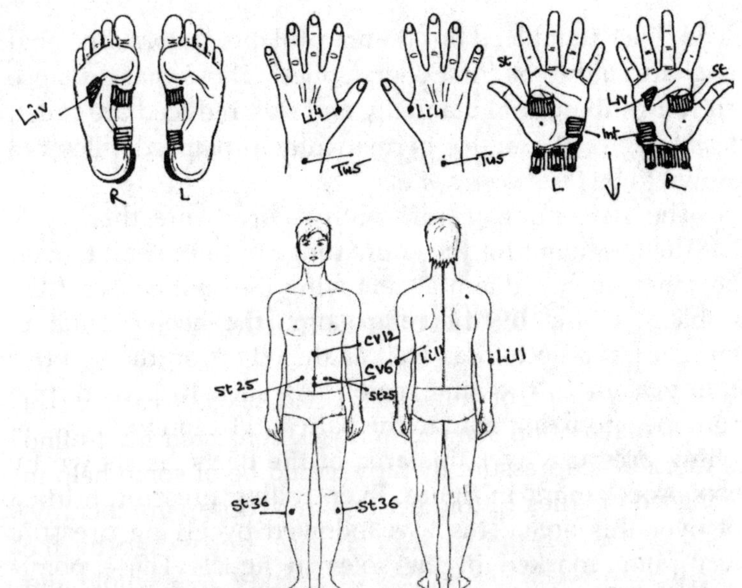

try to make it clear to every new coming patient that we have to take chance for a minimum of three to four days and in case their body starts responding, we can go ahead with the treatment. Hanging on the patient for longer period serves no good purpose.

As scheduled, Mrs. S came on the appointed date. She was about 56 yrs. of age. She was in so much of pain, that after a few sessions, one day she told me, "when I came to you for the first time, I was in so much of pain that I was finding it difficult to resist myself, and I felt like snatching your phone (the moment she came, a patient called for seeking appointment, and I was busy taking the details of his problem(s) and telling you to attend me first of all as I was in so much of pain". It may be understood here that besides the heredity factor, constipation is by and large the root cause of Piles (Hemorrhoids) which could be internal or external in the anal region. Whereas, the internal variety is beneath the anal mucus membrane, external are covered by the skin. Straining causes them to slide downwards and bleed. Piles that bleed but do not prolapse outside the anal canal are said to be 'first degree piles'. Those that prolapse but return to normal manually and stay reduced are called *second degree piles*and& permanently prolapsed piles are known to be *third degree piles*.

The redeeming feature with Acupressure therapy is that the treatment for the entire range of piles shall remain the same, since we aim at removing the root cause of the problem. Going by the reflexology, the heel portion in our soles, the bottom as well as the edges on the anterior side, pertain to the anal region. As such to give respite from the agonizing pain to the patient, I began with giving rolling pressure over this area of the heels, as shown by "xxxxxxxx" mark in figure. Even rolling pressure hurts a lot over this area. This was followed by giving pressure over point marked in the soles in figure. These points pertain to liver, stomach and intestines. The same areas as indicated in figure, depicting palms were also pressed. This was followed by giving pressure over the points shown in figure, over the wrists after giving massage like pressure in the indicated direction, to stimulate the reflexes pertaining to the genitals.

Thereafter, gave pressure on Cv-6. This point is called 'Sea of energy' and is located three finger widths below the naval. Pressure over this point is given after emptying the bladder in lying position with the help of three fingers joined together at an angle of 30 degrees or so. This helps in overcoming constipation.

This has to be followed by giving pressure over St-36 and St-25. Whereas St-36 is located below the knee cap as shown in figure, St-25 is located two thumb widths to the side of the belly button and on back side, on either sides of the spine simultaneously. This point is known for its capability for treating a wide range of intestinal disorders and constipation and is thus considered as a very potent point in acupressure/acupuncture. Medium but firm pressure need to be given over this point to get optimum results. This has to be followed by giving pressure over Cv-12 (Middle stomach), as the name itself suggests, this point is located midway between the belly button and the breast bone. This famous combination of Cv-6; Cv-12 and St-25 which is known as Four doors is extremely beneficial for overcoming any sort of stomach, gastrointestinal disorder including constipation.

Since one of the causes of constipation is excess internal heat, as it dries the stool which makes it too difficult to pass, gave pressure over Tw-5, which is located between 'Ulna' and 'Radius' about three finger widths on the back side of the forehand. This helps in clearing excess heat in the body particularly when pressed in conjunction with Li-4 and Li-11, as has been shown in the figure. Whereas Li-4 clears the excess heat, Li-11 clears the general heat from the body and helps regulate the activity of colon for smooth bowel movement.

The very next day, when Mrs. S came for the sitting, she was happier than expected. Her body had responded very well and reported that though she had pain after passing the stool, yet it was much lesser in intensity as well as duration. The quantum of blood lost was also much less as compared to a day before. She reported that she could see streaks of blood over her stool but it did not fall in drops. Next two sessions provided her further relief and after the third session there was no episode of bleeding. Itching had also gone completely. After around seventh session, she informed that the size of the protrusion outside the anus was also comparatively much reduced. After 11 session she exclaimed while informing that it appears as if air has been taken off from the balloons. In all I gave her 14 sessions. Over the next 10-11 years after her treatment, till I was in her contact, she came twice for just three to four sessions only, on each occasion, when she had a feel of some sort of a relapse, owing to some extra liberty she took with her food habits.

□

Case–16
Infertility

In the year 2003, I was approached by a senior bureaucrat from the Civil Services, saying that his daughter who had been married for about four years was not able to conceive. In our Indian environment, this was a sufficient cause of tension to the parents on both the sides. He wanted to know, if my treatment can bring some relief to them. Needless to mention, it was obvious that they might have done every thing on earth towards the diagnosis as well as treatment before coming for nature cure treatment like acupressure, but they later on shared with me that going by what they had heard about the capability of the therapy and to some extent about my way of handling a patient with absolute transparency, they had come to me with high hope. When asked about any specific abnormality that has been reported after the tests, I was informed that they will bring the reports for a review.

No doubt, not conceiving a child for four years is a cause of concern to the aspiring parents as well as grand parents, but it is also a fact that the more you worry, tension further aggravates the problem. These days, infertility, i.e. inability to conceive is a very common problem. The probable causes could be blockage of the fallopian tubes or some disorder of the uterus or ovaries in the female or low sperm count in the male partner. In any case, both the partners need to be investigated to know where the problem lies and once the causative factor is known, either of the two or both, as

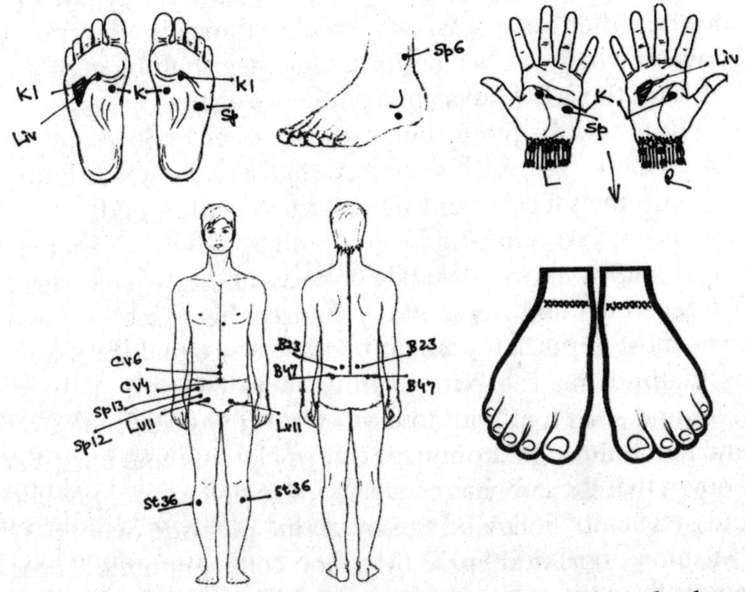

required need to be treated. Further to above, it has also been seen that at times inability to conceive has been found to be due to some sort of imbalances; blockage in the pelvic area, leading to improper menstrual cycle or physical problem with the uterus and fallopian tube that connects the ovaries to the uterus, yet other factor could be deficiency of heat in the pelvis or general lack of blood and energy, etc.

When Mrs. S, aged about 31 yrs., came I told her to set the entire tension/stress aside and have faith in God. She was made to understand that the more tense she will remain it would further delay the process of conception. When she asked me if she could continue with the medication she was getting for more than two years under the care of her gynecologist, along with my treatment, it was made clear to her that I was not going to give her any sort of medication except giving pressure over certain pressure points externally as such she could without any hesitation continue with her medication prescribed by her gynecologist. I further told her that I would be giving her pressure in the first instance for three days consecutively and thereafter thrice a week for two to three months and in between whenever her periods come, we shall be giving a break for those 3-4 days and commence again.

Began with giving her pressure over St-36 point, as shown in the figure. This point strengthens the whole body, tones up the muscles and revitalizes the entire body when pressure is given in conjunction with Sp-6, which lies four finger widths above the ankle bone and is known as 'Three Yin Meeting Point', as shown in figure. This point is known to be most important point to regulate any female problem, as it stimulates the 'Yin' of three meridians, viz. kidney, liver and spleen at the same time and helps flush the Ch'i and blood through the entire body (make sure that once it is known that the lady has conceived, this point should not be pressed at all). Followed this by giving pressure over Sp-12 (Rushing door) and Sp-13 (Mansion cottage) points. These points lie in the groin area in the middle of the crease where the legs join the trunk of the body, as shown in the figure. These two points are considered to be highly effective in overcoming 'Impotency' and 'infertility' problem. They are also known for providing relief in any sort of menstrual irregularity/discomfort.

Next points to be pressed were Cv-4 (Gate Origin) and Cv-6 (Sea of Energy). Both these points lie one below the other, i.e. Cv-6, is located three finger widths below the belly button and Cv-4, is four finger widths below the belly button . Both these points correct imbalances and overcome irregular periods and impotency. Cv-6 also strengthens the overall reproductive system. The patient was told to press this point for 10 to 15 days every day even on the days she was not supposed to come for the treatment and thereafter every alternate day till she conceived even when the treatment was over (not to be pressed during her periods). Further, I pressed B-23 and B-47, these points are located in the middle of the waist as shown in the figure. These two points have a positive effect on sexual reproductivity, impotence, and premature ejaculation. Next point pressed was K-1, known as bubbling springs, is located on the sole of the foot in the centre between the two pads. Also gave pressure on Lv-11, a point known as 'Yin corner', is located two thumbs widths below the upper edge of the pubic bone, as shown in the figure. This too helps overcome infertility.

Besides giving pressure over the aforesaid points, also give pressure over the wrists and feet as shown in the figure. Whereas the points marked '*' over the wrists and below the ankle to stimulate the sex organs, as also the area marked 'xxxxxxx' help overcome any sort of blockage in the fallopian tubes. Within a year, Mrs. S was blessed with a son, by the grace of God. She came to me for her Cervical problem about six months back from Dubai and I was pleased to meet her two sons who accompanied her and have now grown up to 11 and 9 yrs of age.

□

Case–17
Hypertension

In the year 1999, when I went to visit a patient suffering from paralysis, I forgot to take my mobile phone with me. In my absence, my wife who was a diabetic and was also undergoing treatment for heart problem as she had suffered angina pain about two years ago noticed that her blood pressure had shot to 168/107. A matter of co-incidence, her brother came to our home in some connection and since I was not home, in a panic he took her to Dr. R.M.L. Hospital, where she was admitted in 'Emergency'. As it happened to be a Sunday, they had only skeletal staff at that point of time. When I came back home, my younger son informed me about the episode and that she has been taken to the hospital where she is in emergency ward. I went to the hospital and was informed that her blood pressure has been found to be 170/110 at the time of admission and as such they have admitted her for management and observation. On further enquiry from the patient, I was told that she had been there for about 30-40 minutes but no medication has been given to her, as an accident case had come and obviously, the entire attention of the Senior Resident as well as the Intern was diverted to that more serious case.

The symptoms of hypertension include a dull headache, nose bleed (at times), dizziness, heaviness in the head, etc. and the causative factors could be faulty eating habits, mental stress, excessive physical strain, lack of exercising, alcohol consumption/smoking, inadequate sleep, etc.,

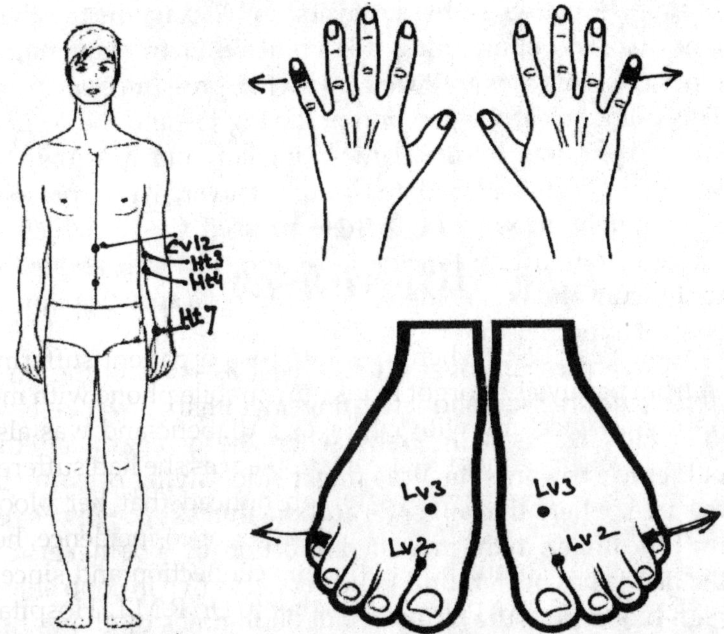

but all I could see in the present situation was that she was complaining of heaviness in her head which was attributable to disturbed sleep the previous night as *'Devi Jagran'* was going on in the neighborhood and the sound of the speakers might have kept her awake as well as the high blood pressure she had at the moment.

In terms of acupuncture/acupressure, it could be caused due to excess of 'Yang' or excess of phlegm or damp. Such a deficiency may occur in kidney or liver which control the circulation of Ch'i. However, whatever be the cause, uncontrolled blood pressure can lead to other serious problems like damage to the kidney(s); brain hemorrhage; eye problem or even paralysis.

Since the doctors on duty were busy, I started giving her pressure. First of all I gave pressure over Lv-3 point which lies between the big and the second toe on top of the foot, as shown in the figure. This point tonifies the liver and the flow of Ch'i in the liver meridian, as one of the prominent causes of hypertension is blockage in the liver meridian and stimulating this point removes stagnation/ blockage. This was followed by giving pressure over Lv-2. This point lies at the junction of the big toe and the second toe. It is known by the name 'Xingjian' and is known to stimulate 'Yin' and Sedate 'Yang' of liver, when pressed in combination with Lv-3. Also pressed Cv-12, which is located along the midline of the abdomen, a little above the umbilicum and is considered to be almost a specific point to control hypertension.

Gave pressure over Ht-7 as well as Ht-3 on the little finger side precisely about two finger widths below the elbow joint. Ht-7 lies just at the crease where the lower arm and the palm meet towards the little finger side. Giving pressure in the area, where the nail ends and the thin skin begins, over the little finger, in the indicated direction, over both feet and the hands has been found to be very effective in controlling high blood pressure. After about 30 minutes of giving her acupressure, I requested the doctor on duty, who had by that time become a bit free, to get her blood pressure rechecked. He told me that they have yet to start her medication and he saw no reason to recheck B.P. When I insisted, he asked the sister on duty to check the blood pressure of my patient and when the sister on duty informed him that the B.P. has come down to 140/95, he did not believe her and went to check himself, as he told that he had himself rechecked her blood pressure when sister on duty reported 170/110 at the time of admission. When he too found that the pressure has come down, he started questioning the patient (to know the cause of sudden fall in her blood pressure as to what had happened, or did she take any medicine on her own while in the hospital). I introduced myself to him and told him that since they were busy attending the accident case, I had given her acupressure therapy and the down fall was the outcome of the therapy. We kept the patient in the hospital for another an hour and when the pressure did not go up again, I requested the doctor to relieve her on my request and brought her home. Later on it came to light that the rise was a due to stress owing to disturbed sleep as also because the patient had not exercised due restraint in her food intake during the dinner in the party and to add to the problem, she had forgotten to take the medicine that night as she did not come home immediately after the dinner and sat there to attend the *Jagran* for quite some time.

For some days the above pressure points were pressed and check was kept over the trend of her blood pressure to rule out repetition of the incidence. She was advised to make sure that under no circumstances she should miss the prescribed dose of medicine.

□

Case–18
Electrocution

It was in the year 1992, when one of my friends, Mr. P, aged about 45 yrs. while working in his office during the rainy season, got an electric shock when he tried to attach some electrical cord in one of the switch points. The news spread as it was a panic situation and a fellow worker came running to my chamber asking for help to carry him to the nearby hospital. While I sent for the driver to get the car ready for carrying Mr. P to the hospital, I thought to give him first aid and went to his room. To the utter surprise of all the onlookers, within two to three minutes, Mr. P who had gone unconscious and was not even able to raise his hands, opened his eyes and sat down. On being told that we are going to shift him to the nearest hospital, he said I am perfectly all right and there is no need to go to the hospital. He requested me to give another round of pressure points, as he was aware that I give acupressure treatment. Encouraged by his body response, we decided to wait for another couple of minutes, sent for coffee for us and in the meantime coffee was brought and it was finished, acupressure over the following points was given and within 20-25 minutes or so he was perfectly all right. Still I insisted that we should visit the hospital to rule out any after-effect and accompanied him to the Dr. R.M.L. Hospital, New Delhi, where the doctors after examining him found nothing abnormal with him and sent him back. Rather they wanted to know what

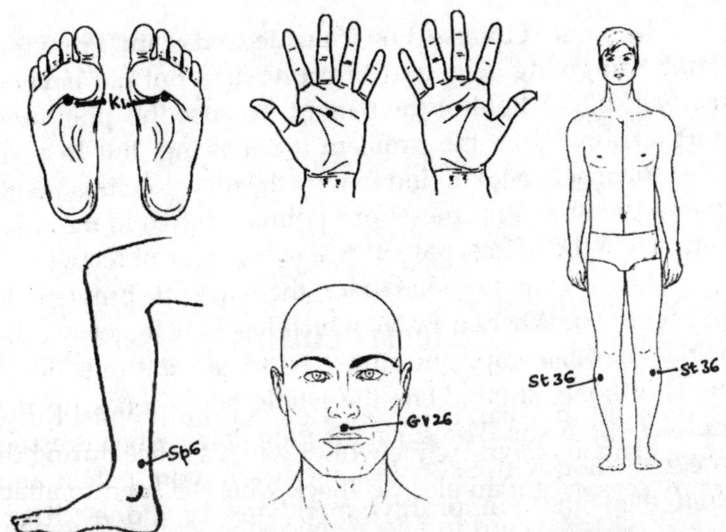

were the pressure points pressed so that they could be tried over such in coming cases in future for their benefit.

The pressure points pressed were K-1, this point lies between the pads of the soles below the big toe and the pad formed on the other side of the little finger. This point which is known by the name 'Bubbling Springs' has been found to be worth its name and surprisingly acts so fast in this sort of a situation that it boosts your energy levels to the heights and the patient, who at times might even loose consciousness as a result of the shock, regains consciousness within a few seconds by giving deep pressure over this point three times, just for the duration of 10 seconds, on each occasion.

On the similar lines, pressure in the palms should also be given over the pressure point as shown in figure. This point pertains to the area of solar plexus in our body and the simplest way to locate this point is to hold the palm facing the sky, we come across many lines in our palm but out of the three prominent lines in our palms, look for the line in the middle of the palm, imagine where it shall cross the middle line in case we extend the middle finger towards our wrist.

The point of intersection is the desired point. Press this point also giving deep and firm pressure, but not beyond the pain thresh hold of the patient, because this point will hurt terribly when the problem it persisting. But to your utter surprise, you will find that by the time you finish with giving pressure over these four points, i.e. two in the soles and two in the palms, patient will show signs of recovery.

After giving pressure over these points press St-36 and Sp-6 too. Whereas St-36, which lies four finger widths below the knee cap, one finger width on the outside of the shin bone, strengthens the whole body, tones up the muscles , Sp-6, the 'Three Yin Meeting Point' when pressed in conjunction with St-36, becomes even more potent and strengthens the 'Yin' of three meridians, i.e. kidney; liver, and spleen at the same time. Helps flush the Ch'i and blood through the body and thus does the rest of the job to bring out the patient from the electric shock. Finally, I gave pressure over Gv-26 point which is located on the upper lip in the middle of the centre of our nose. This point is very frequently used as a 'First aid revival point', which helps overcome fainting, dizziness, etc.

In a similar incident, my younger son, aged 25 years, suffered an electric shock from the room cooler, while filling water in its water tank, in the year 2001. A tall and healthy young man who has a robust health, as he used to resort to daily exercises. After getting the electric shock, his hand hung in the air and was not able to lift his right hand at all. His eyes had become blood red. Somehow he had managed to get his hand free from the grip. As he shouted, I rushed for his help as fortunately I was home. Looking into his condition, I lost no time in deciding to take him to the Safdarjung hospital.

However, the next moment I recalled Mr. P's case a few years ago and decided to spend 2-3 minutes with him at home trying to revive him. Gave pressure as narrated above, and after about just two minutes of giving him the therapy, I asked him, if he could hold my hand? He said let me try and he held my hand and pressed with so much force that I had to tell him to hold my hand softly. Soon, within half an hour or so the color of his eye balls became normal and when I asked him to come for a checkup to the hospital, he commented... What for?

Here in this context, a word of caution... Electric injury is caused by the passage of electric current. The tissues of the body being moist and salty are a good conductor of electricity. Dry skin provides a high resistance. Persons in the bath rooms are more at a risk. Similarly, AC is more risky than DC current.

The first thing one can and should do is to break the person's contact with the source of electricity, without directly touching them. You can also try giving first-aid treatment using the aforesaid pressure points, but make sure that you are giving first aid only. Do not assume the role of a doctor till you are fully confident and find that the patient has recovered completely and is talking like a normal person. Still it would be better in case expert advise of a professional medical consultant is taken to rule out any side effect.

□

Case--19
Migraine

I recall of a case of migraine and cervical spondylosis, I handled in the year 2001. A female about 38 years of age, a teacher by profession, called me to take appointment at around 8.30 pm and said she wanted to come immediately as she had an attack of migraine. I told her that it may not be possible to attend her at that time since I already had two patients in the waiting and that I would not be able to do justice to her, in case even if I give her appointment. I told her to come next day in the morning at 8.00 am. Next day when she came, while taking the history of her case, I was informed that she has been suffering from this problem for almost 7-8 years. She had undergone treatment from doctors from many streams of medicine and she admitted that she did get partial relief from Allopathy and Ayurveda treatment but the relief was short lived and the moment she stopped treatment, she again started getting bouts of migraine headache. On being asked why she did not try Homeopathy, she said she did try and got some relief there too but unfortunately, the doctor attending her left the city along with her parents as such the treatment could not be continued. Presently, finding no other option she had taken recourse to the conventional stream, i.e. she was under the treatment of an Allopathic Physician, however, she said that she wanted to stop taking pain killers as she had heard a lot about the side effect of the medicines she has been taking. She also reported that she has noticed that there is some

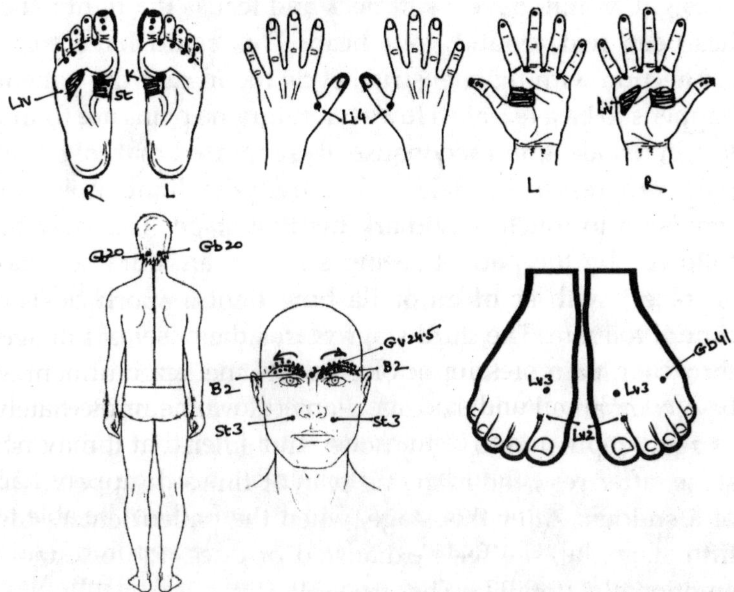

connection between her pain, periods and the exams, in the schools. About the nature of her headache, she informed that it throbs, it bangs, and it squeezes. It begins early in the morning, with intense pain in one side of the head or behind the eyes. At times it spreads to the entire head, she is not able to bear light or sound at all. Does not want to talk to any one. On being asked about the duration of the pain, she commented most of the times it goes on for three to four days and only occasionally it settles after seven or eight hours in case some how she is able to sleep.

In this context, it may be of interest to note that migraine is an extremely painful medical situation, in which the patient suffers throbbing and pulsating sort of pain, which settles, generally, in one side of the head. This can happen at any age. In case your pain persists for three to four days, prevents you from doing your day-to-day routine work, headache comes like a sudden 'explosion', you experience weakness in you limbs or feel disoriented, difficulty in speaking, experience problems with your eyesight, vomit, have a stiff neck and feel as if a tight band has been tied around your head. This could have some connection with the menstrual cycle too in case the patient happens to be a female. However, migraine pains are found less in female after menopause. It is reported that migraine pain progresses in stages. Sensitivity to light, noise or repulsion to touch may mark the first stage. This may be followed by the patient seeing a sort of an 'aura' around an object with sparkles or flashing lights, which he/she cannot tolerate. The third stage marks the onset of intense, throbbing pain settling in one side of the head. This may be accompanied with nausea, diarrhea, weakness as well as extreme repulsion to light, noise, and smells. In the fourth stage, after rest, the migraine pain at times disappears all of a sudden. After this stage, when the patient enters the fifth stage, he/she feels exhausted or does not feel stable emotionally, not in his/her true self.

Since acupressure therapy helps in removing the root cause of the problem, i.e. pain in this case by relaxing the muscles, releasing blocked flow in the energy channels, relieving tension and improving the supply of 'Oxygen' to the brain cells, the following schedule was followed: Started with giving pressure over all the sinus points over the finger tips in both the feet and the palms as also pressing the brain point located on the top of the big toe as well as the thumbs as shown in figure. Stimulating these points improves circulation of the blood to the brain and as a consequence thereof improves the supply of oxygen to the brain. Also stimulate the pressure points pertaining to the cervical region, pituitary, lymph nodes, stomach, liver, kidneys, spine, and adrenals as shown in the figure referred to above. Also pinch around the points marked by the dots over the eye brows in figure, these point hurt a lot on being pinched, but have been found to be of immense importance in overcoming problems, e.g. migraine, insomnia, fits, etc.

By virtue of their stress relieving capabilities, these pressure points have earned the name of 'Stress Buster Points'.

This was followed by giving pressure over St-3, a point known by the name 'Facial Beauty' and is located at the bottom of the cheek bone, in line with the pupil . Stimulating this point results into decongestion of head, eye strain, and headache. Next points pressed were B-2 (Drilling Bamboo) that lies over the bridge of the nose between the eye brows. It relieves the eye fatigue, strain, and headache as well as Gv-24.5, the 'Third Eye' which is located between the eyebrows as shown in the figure. This balances the functions of the pituitary gland and relieves headache as well as eye strain.

Here after, press Li-4 (Adjoining Valley), this is known for its ability to relieve pain and help restore the flow of Ch'i through the body. It also helps into elimination of toxins through bowels, removes stagnation of Ch'i too. Pregnant women should not be given pressure over this point. Next points pressed were Gb-20 and Gb-41. Gb-20 is known by the name 'Gates of Consciousness', is located below the base of the skull, only mild pressure should be given over these points simultaneously on both sides. It helps in overcoming the stiffness in the region of neck. It is also helpful in eliminating wind and cold. Gb-41 is located between the fourth and fifth metatarsal bones on the top of the foot, as shown in figure. This point restores the flow of Ch'i and is helpful in mitigating migraine pain. Finally, before ending the session, I pressed Lv-3, which lies on the top of the feet between the big toe and the second toe about two finger widths above Lv-2 which lies at the junction of big toe and the second toe. It tonifies the liver and the flow of Ch'i through the liver meridian, an organ considered to be most powerful organ for 'detoxification. It improves the functioning of the gall bladder besides relieving nausea, vomiting, etc.

During the course of treatment, the patient informed that she also examines the Board exam copies as also she was responsible to get even the mid-year exams in the school conducted. In the process, she had to undergo lots of strain after the exams were over, as she was required to handle thousands of answer sheets. Accordingly, I had given her pressure points to cover both cervical as well as for her migraine problem. The treatment lasted for about 14 sessions in all and the patient who kept in touch with me for many years, since every time before she was required to handle huge number of answer sheets for checking, she had made it a point to take 3-4 sessions as 'preventive' treatment and had never complained of any severe pain thereafter. No doubt, at times, she felt that migraine pain might trigger, but since I had explained her the points to be pressed and how to press them, as and when she had the slightest inkling of getting the migraine triggered, she used to press those points and later reported that either the pain does not come at all or if at all it comes, the intensity is too low and the duration is also comparatively too less and it subsides without taking any medicine just by taking rest. Gradually, the incidence of even such minor episodes also kept decreasing.

□

Case–20
Loss of Voice/Sensation in Lower Limbs Due to Fall

During the year 2009, when I used to go to the GTB Hospital, UCMS, Delhi for taking OPD's thrice a week, one day an Asstt. Nursing Supdt. of the hospital, who had also undergone training from me, telephoned me to inform that one of her relations' daughter had a fall from the cot on a Friday night and since then she is neither able to move her lower limbs nor she is able to speak after the fall. She had been admitted to the hospital two days back on a Saturday and has been undergoing treatment there for the past two days. Since I used to visit the hospital on Monday, Wednesday, and Friday, she requested me to pay a visit in the ward before going to my OPD since it may be difficult for me to come out before afternoon once I enter the OPD. I agreed and told her to be present there when I come so that I tell her what to do on the days I will not be able to visit.

Accordingly, around 9.30 am, I phoned her to reach the ward where the patient Miss. V, aged about 16-17 years, was admitted. I found that besides what had been reported over phone by the ANS, the girl also had some effect over her mouth (i.e. a mild attack of 'facial paralysis' too), besides loss of voice and sensation/strength in the lower limbs. My schedule of plan comprised of the following pressure points.

Began with giving pressure over Gb-2 and Gb-12 points. Whereas Gb-2 lies in front of the ear at the joint of

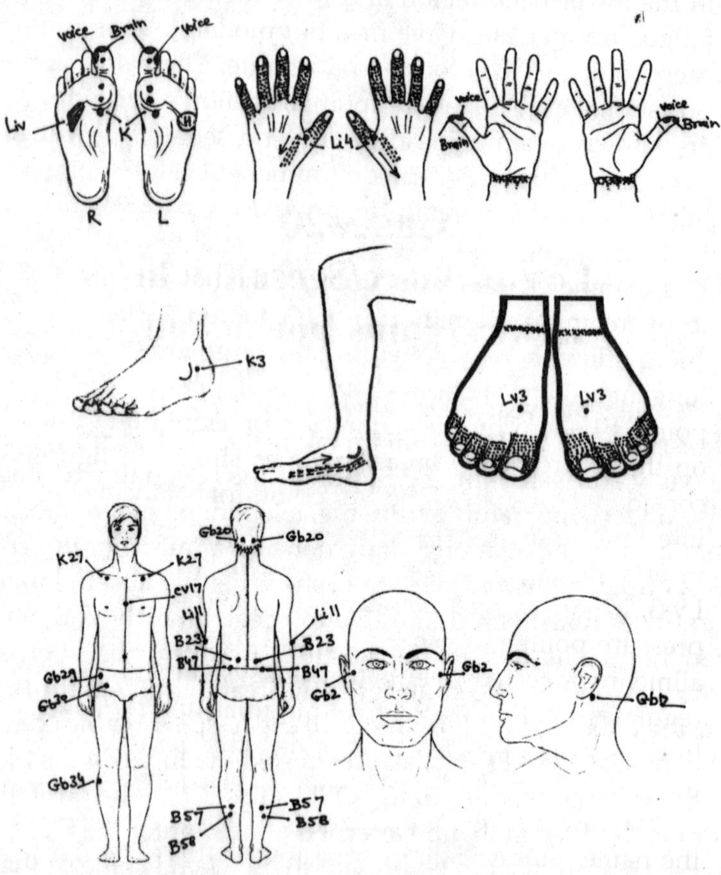

the jaw, Gb-12 is located in the depression behind the ears, below the mastoid bone, as shown in figure, both these points are almost specific to treat 'facial paralysis'. Next, I pressed Gb-20 which is known by the name 'Gates of Consciousness' and is located in the hollow below the base of the skull, and has been considered to be highly beneficial in overcoming the stiffness in the region of the neck as well as in eliminating the wind and cold present, thereby restoring the energy imbalance(s), if any in the kidney and bladder meridians. Also press B-23 and B-47 points whose location is shown in figure these points are useful in providing relief in the lower back region and in reducing muscle tension, fatigue trauma, etc., gave firm but moderate pressure over each point for 30 seconds to a minute. Thereafter applied pressure over K-27 and K-3 points, as shown in figure. They are known to stimulate the 'Yin' and sedate the 'Yang' of liver and kidneys. For maximum benefit ask the patient to inhale and exhale breath deeply. Also gave pressure over Li-4 (Adjoining Valley) and Li-11 (Crooked Pond). Whereas Li-4 eliminates the toxins through the bowels, it is helpful in overcoming stagnation in Ch'i too. Li-11 helps restore energy flow thereby benefiting the large intestines and the lung meridians. Followed by this, I pressed CV-17, this point is known by the name 'Sea of Tranquility', this lies on the centre of the breast bone as shown in figure, and considered to be one of the best points for balancing the small intestines and the heart meridian and is extremely useful in establishing 'emotional' balance in our body. Pressing Lv-3, a point which has been found to be most essential pressure point and can be pressed for help in almost any ailment connected to either of the systems in our body. It regulates and tonifies the liver meridian and the 'Ch'i in the liver meridian besides overcoming the damage caused to the gallbladder and liver meridians, besides detoxification.

Follow this by giving pressure over Gb-34, (known by the name 'Sunny Side of the Mountain', this point lies in the depression below the bony prominence on the lateral side of the knee. This points dispels wind, clears damp heat and stimulates the liver's 'Yin'. Liver nourishes the joints, mobility of the joint, muscular strain is improved by giving pressure over this point. Gb-30 known as 'Jumping Circle', and Gb-29 are other important points, as shown in the figure, are very useful for relieving hip joint problem besides stimulating circulation in the entire leg and low back. Since the muscle in this part of the body is sufficiently thicker, in case you are not able to reach this point with the help of your thumbs (one over the other to exert double pressure),

pressure can be given with the help of your elbow, but very cautiously. Also press B-57 (Support the Mountain) and B-58, as shown in figure, to get relief in leg pain and also stiffness in that area.

Since Paralysis is an ailment which directly or indirectly involves the entire range of systems in our body, as such while trying to overcome this problem, all the pressure points discussed above need to be stimulated at least for first five to seven days every day and thereafter depending upon the body response of the patient, whereas pressure over one set of the points can be given on day one and the same over the second set of points can be given on the other day to get maximum relief. Needless to say, besides the above pressure points, pressure should also be given over the reflex points pertaining to all major organs in the body e.g. brain, nervous system, heart, liver, lungs, Endocrine system (i.e. pituitary, adrenals, thyroid; para-thyroid, pancreas, lymphatic system, etc.) at least 2-3 times a week as explained above. Also gave pressure on the inner side of the big toe as well as thumbs at the shaded portion as shown in the figure. Giving pressure over this area yields very good results in restoration of lost voice. Deep pressure needs to be given over this area.

The patient responded very well and to my utter surprise, around 6.00 pm, the same day, I got a call from the hospital that the girl has started speaking, though the voice was not very clear yet people around her could make out what she was trying to say. Within five days her voice quality had barely 20% distortion and more than 50% of the facial paralysis part, i.e. the twist of her mouth towards one side had returned towards normalcy. The girl was discharged from the hospital in seven days and her treatment continued for yet another month or so.

□

Case–21
Sinusitis

In the year 2007, a friend of my son who worked in a senior position in one of the multi national companies approached me for his Sinus problem. He told me that he had been suffering this problem for more than 12 years and had undergone treatment at many places and finally the doctors had advised him to go for surgery. But he was not willing to go for that option, since he had spoken to many persons who had undergone surgery, but found that most of them were not too happy since of and on they kept suffering even after the surgery. I told him that there is no harm in trying treatment under acupressure therapy. His treatment was taken up.

Before I discuss the points pressed, it may be of interest for the readers to know that sinuses are the air filled spaces on either side of the nose on our face. They are sort of tiny hollow compartments in the head leading from nose, behind our eyes and cheek bone to the forehead. Once these tiny openings are obstructed, the mucus produced there cannot be drained out. This results into accumulation of fluids in these cavities which results into heaviness and pain. The problem gets further aggravated since the openings that drain our maxillary sinuses are located very inconveniently, i.e. upside down. These passages close when the tissues swell because of allergens, smoke or viruses. Such infections can result into a sort of benign nasal growth known as 'Polyp'.

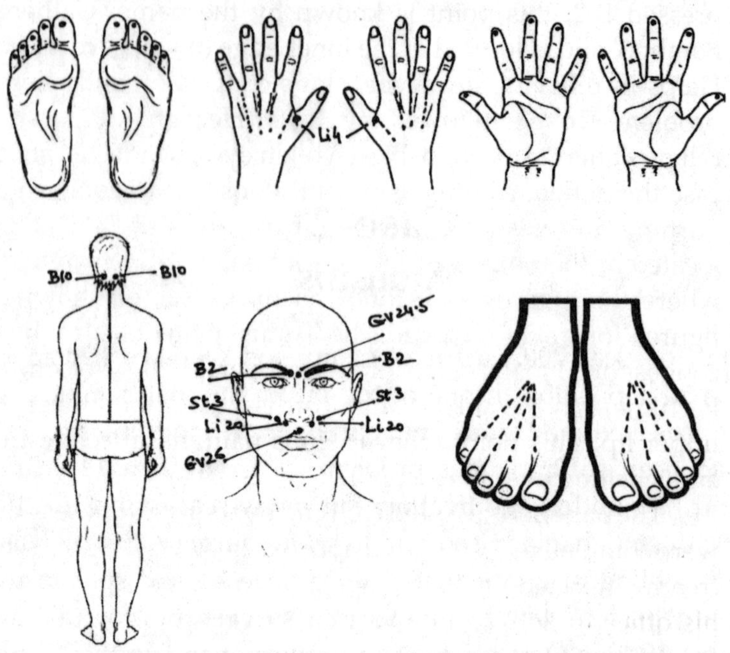

In the instant case, the following schedule was followed. Began with giving pressure over the sinus points that are located over the tip of all the fingers, below brain points in the big toes and the thumbs as shown in figure. This was followed by giving pressure in the channels shown by the dotted lines over the dorsum of the feet and back of the palms. This was followed by giving pressure over Li-4, 'Adjoining Valley'. This point is considered to be one of the most effective pressure points to overcome headache and relax muscles. It also balances the flow of energy in the lower and upper part of the body. Pregnant women should not press this point, as it may cause miscarriage. Next important point to be pressed is Gv-24.5, this point is known as 'The Third Eye', where the eyebrows and the bridge of the nose meet. This point balances the pituitary gland which corrects the functioning of thyroid gland and removes 'sinus' congestion, headache, and eyestrain. Then pressed B-2, this point is known by the name 'Gathered Bamboo' and is located at the inner edge of your eye socket. Helps in relieving headache, sinus congestion and allergy problem. To be followed by B-10 (Heavenly Pillars), it relieves allergic reaction, like swollen eyes, headache, etc. In case the patient complains of stuffy nose, head congestion, burning and swelling over the eyes, press St-3, which is located at the bottom of the cheek bone a little away from where the nostrils end, followed by Gv-26, as shown in figure, for relief in headache, sinus pain as also head congestion. Finally, give pressure over Li-20 (Welcoming Perfume), on the side of the nostrils where they meet the upper lip. This point relieves sinus pain, nasal congestion and swelling over the face.

The patient responded well and by the time four sessions were completed, he reported approx. 25-30% relief. In all his treatment lasted for 16 sessions. Thereafter, he invited me to his office to deliver an" Awareness Talk on Acupressure" for the benefit of senior and middle management.

□

Case–22
Internal Bleeding

An old colleague of mine aged about 57 yrs. phoned me one day to inform that he is admitted in AIIMS Hospital, since he had been bleeding intermittently for about 24 hours off and on before he got himself admitted. The cause of bleeding was not known. He confirmed that he was not suffering from 'piles' or any other known disease which might be responsible for this sort of intermittent bleeding. As a courtesy, I told him that I shall be visiting him during the visiting hours in the evening.

When I reached him, I found that he was too much worried. He had lost his wife only a few months back, as such he was being looked after by his bhabhiji. Since I had gone only as a visitor, while chatting I came to know that after admission in the hospital, since he was admitted after 2.30 pm on a Saturday, being half day, he was being kept there under observation only. He told me that he was not getting due attention as expected. Next day being Sunday, he was all the more worried. Casually, he asked me in case he can be helped any way by acupressure therapy. I told him that there was no harm in applying pressure, in case his bleeding could be stopped. Frankly speaking, till that day (this episode took place in the year 1993 if I can recall correctly), I had not come across any case of internal bleeding of this sort, wherein the cause was not known. I had handled minor cases of children hurting their lips with their teeth after a fall while playing which ends up in bleeding or

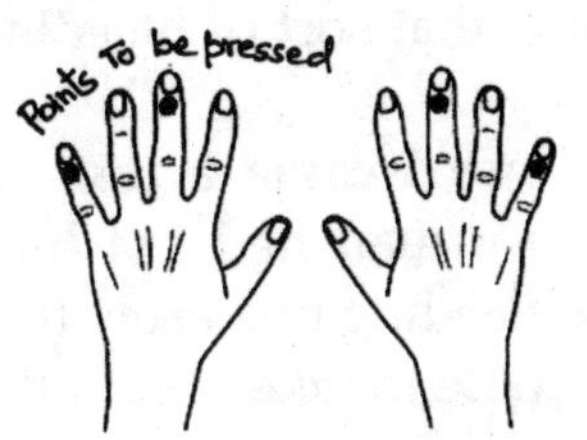

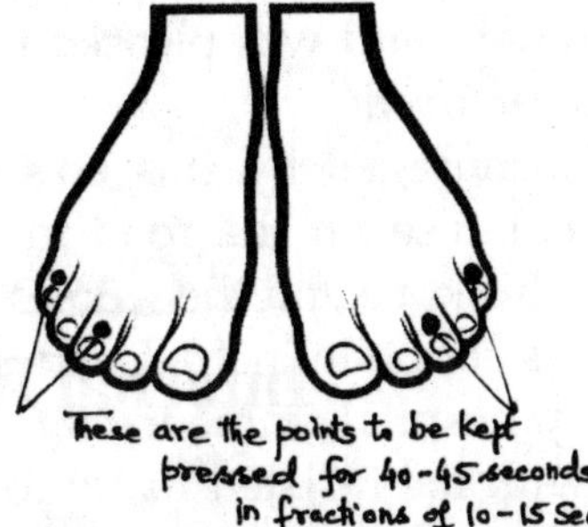

some minor accident cases in which I could help stopping the bleeding by applying pressure over certain reflex points and also adopting the means, the old timers used to apply, e.g. applying turmeric or sugar in the area of the cut, which generally leads to stopping the oozing out blood from the point of injury.

I started applying pressure over the little finger and the middle fingers of the left hand and the left feet, at the junction where thin skin over the finger ends and the nail starts. This is the reflex area where pressure is given to control blood pressure, the area to be pressed have been shown in figure. Since the process required four points to be pressed at the same time, I requested his bhabhi to help me by holding the pressure points over his hand while I held the same points over his feet, for about 30 to 45 seconds. After giving pressure on the left limbs, we switched over to giving pressure over the right hand and feet, over the same area as on the left side. Here too pressure was given for 30-45 seconds. I repeated the entire process for the second time after a gap of about 15 minutes. While coming back, I told his bhabhi, who was going to stay back with him in the hospital, to repeat the process one by one on all the four limbs once again in the night and again the next day morning. The next day when I phoned him to know how he was , he informed that after he was given pressure by me twice and thereafter by his bhabhi repeated the same two times, the bleeding stopped and as such he asked the doctors to relieve him and he has come home. I kept in touch with him for more than seven days and was pleased to know that sort of bleeding never recurred.

Encouraged by this episode, once I came across an accident case on the road in which a man had got hurt below his knee and the wound was bleeding profusely (the cut was about an inch). I told the people to take him to the nearby hospital immediately, but one of my juniors who was with me insisted to try for a minute if we could help him. Pressure as explained above was given by both of us. Since the cut in this case was clearly over the right knee, we gave pressure only on the right side and surprisingly the oozing of the blood stopped within no time, say in 45-50 seconds. Thereafter, his wound was dressed after cleaning carefully after about half an hour, by which time the blood had clotted properly.

The inference is that acupressure therapy can be applied as a first aid too, even in an emergent situation, of course with an open mind that we are not here to prove any thing but to provide relief to the patient in the best of his interest. Under no circumstances, time should be wasted on such accident cases where the opening of the cut/wound is so wide open or deep that it may required stitching. In other cases of minor injuries in case you feel the we can get the results within a minute or two, it is fine, otherwise recourse to conventional medicine should be taken.

□

Case–23
Asthama of Long Standing

Somewhere in the year 1995, I happened to attend the case of a person, Mr. V, who used to run a printing press. He was about 55 years of age and I was told he has been suffering from asthma for more than 25 years. Obviously, his problem was partially aggravated due to his profession too since in those days most of the printing job was done on off set press in which printing process involved use of lots of chemicals, which emit pungent gases like ammonia. I was supposed to give home visits to the patient.

Here in this context, let us try to analyse and understand the symptoms and causes of this problem. The problem is marked by shortness of breath, particularly while exhaling, wheezing, tightness in the chest compels the patient to sit and lean forward in his effort to use his neck/chest to help him breath. The patient coughs up mucus, he has spasm in the walls of the bronchial tubes, air passage becomes narrow. The causative factors could be dust, smoke, pollen, smog, or some environmental pollutants as well. Allergies are also known to be the prominent causative factor behind this sort of an ailment. Non-allergens can also trigger bronchial spasms, the common factors being rigorous exercising, emotional stress, cold air, viral infections or even the side effect of some medication. Heredity factor is also among one of the prime causative factors in such ailments.

The treatment commenced and after attending the patient in the evening around 7.30 pm, I came back home. However, before I could reach home, a call had been received

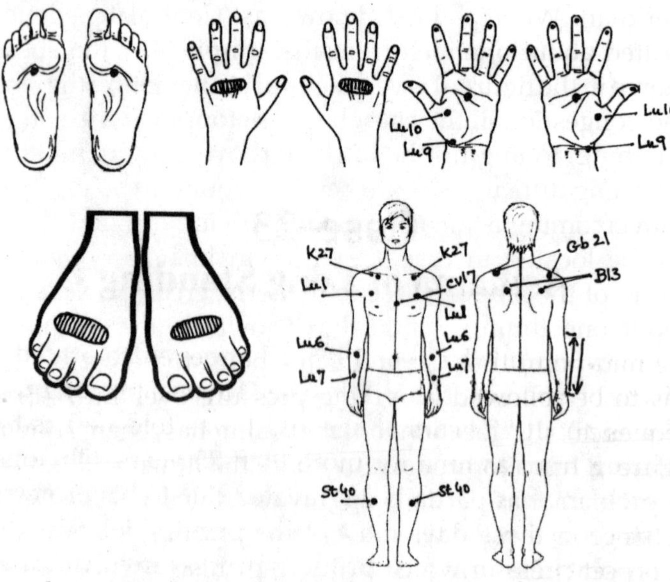

from the patient's home that after taking the treatment, the condition of the patient has worsened. I was surprised by the news since I had never heard of or came across any case in which the condition of the patient might have deteriorated after giving the therapy. It may be a different matter that the treatment may not suit a particular person or he/she does not get immediate relief. Any way, I had no option but to rush back to the patients house and when I reached there, I found that the gentleman was oozing out so much of cough that he and his family members got scared. When I asked him, why he does not want the accumulated cough to be thrown out of his body and was he not feeling lighter? He remarked that no doubt he was feeling lighter and was able to breathe comparatively easily, but they got scared at the sight of so much of cough. I sat there for about two hours, gave pressure over certain points to calm him down and asked him to take his dinner in my presence. After he fell asleep, I came back home.

The following was the plan of treatment adopted. Commenced with giving pressure over Lu-1, Lu-6, Lu-7,

Lu-9, and Lu-10, all the aforesaid points pertain to the lung meridian. Whereas Lu-1, known as 'Central Residence' is located about one inch from the armpit over the chest, as shown in the figure, it is very helpful in alleviating the tension and congestion in the chest besides stopping wheezing and coughing, toning up the lungs and overcoming all kind of breathing difficulties. Lu-6 has been found to be very useful in overcoming acute condition involving lungs. This point can be located in case we draw an imaginary line from centre of the elbow crease to the wrist crease, divide it and about one thumb width above towards the elbow from the mid-point thus arrived is the point to be pressed. This has to be followed by giving pressure over Lu-7 (Broken Sequence). Its location on the palm has been shown in figure. It has a tonifying effect over the lungs and improves their functioning. Next point I pressed was Lu-9, which lies in the groove at the wrist fold, below the base of the thumb. This point helps in coughing out the phlegm from the lungs, making the breathing easier, followed by giving pressure over Lu-10, known by the name 'Fish Border', as shown in the figure. It relieves breathing, coughing and helps sooth swollen throat.

After this, I gave pressure over the 'lung Associated Point', i.e. B-13, which lies between the spine and the scapula blade, as shown in figure. This point relieves asthma, coughing, and sneezing. Followed by giving pressure over Cv-17, directly over the breast bone. Whereas for men this point can be located at the level of nipples between the fourth and fifth ribs, for women it lies about three finger widths above the breast bone. Use tips of three fingers joined together to press this point. In case B-13 and Cv-17 are pressed consecutively, their effect is more beneficial. This combination has to be used in chronic cases of asthma. K-27 was the next point to be pressed, as has been shown (below the breast bone) in the figure. It provides relief in breathing, chest congestion, overcoming stress in the region of the chest. Next point was Gb-21, which is known as

'Shoulder Well', as shown, i.e. mid way between the outer edge of the shoulder and the neck. To end the session, gave pressure over St-40 point. This point lies half way between the ankle bone on the outside of the foot and the centre of the knee cap. In case you find that cough and mucus is accumulated in the lungs, pressing this point helps throw out that phlegm and clear the congestion. While pressing these points, ask the patient to take slow but deep breaths to get better effect.

Pressure over all the aforesaid points can be given for the first three or four days regularly, thereafter, some of them can be omitted in one session and taken up in the next session by omitting certain other points pressed in the previous session. Also give pressure over the sinus, lungs, solar plexus, bronchial reflexes on the dorsal portion of the feet and the hands, as also over the entire lung meridian over the fore arm, on the thumb side, starting from wrist to the elbow joint, as shown in the figure, up and down motion giving massage like pressure. Giving pressure over this area provides instant relief from congestion and breathlessness.

By the time, the fifth session was over, the patient reported around 25% relief. He was advised to reduce taking puffs in consultation with his physician. Mr. V informed that he had already cut down taking puffs just after third session and nowadays he was taking puffs only three times a day whereas before starting the treatment, he used to take five to six puffs at times. Still I asked him to do all this in consultation with his physician. By the time 12 sessions were given he brought down taking puffs only once in the night, as a precaution and had resorted to taking puff only SOS. In all 17 sessions were given. Thereafter, while stopping his treatment, I marked a chart of pressure points to be given and gave it to him with the advice to take pressure at the onset of change of weather himself even in case he had no problem, since that is the time when asthma triggers.

□

Case–24
Depression

Somewhere in the year 1998-99, Mr. J, aged 53 yrs., was introduced to me by one of my old patients. This gentleman was suffering from severe depression for more than four years and has been under the treatment of a senior psychiatrist. By profession, the patient was into business. His only son who came along with the patient, told me in private that his father had suffered heavy losses in business. He was robbed by the 'Blacks' in the States, but fortunately his life was spared. Here in the country, his business partner whom he treated just like his brother and, while away to the States, had even given the cheque signing powers had also ditched him and this man was a totally shattered person. He had even tried to commit suicide once. With a patient of this sort and the circumstances around him, there was nothing new in his behavior.

In this context, at the outset, let us understand that in every one's life, at times the things seem not happening the way we expect or plan, every thing seems to be going out of hands. In such circumstances, whereas one set of people do not loose self-confidence and keep struggling boldly, the other set of people take things to their heart, become extremely sad. No charm is left in their life. Such people tend to focus only on negative side of life. The causes could be external as above or biological caused by chemical imbalances in the system and psychological. At times, in case you keep on controlling your anger or emotions for

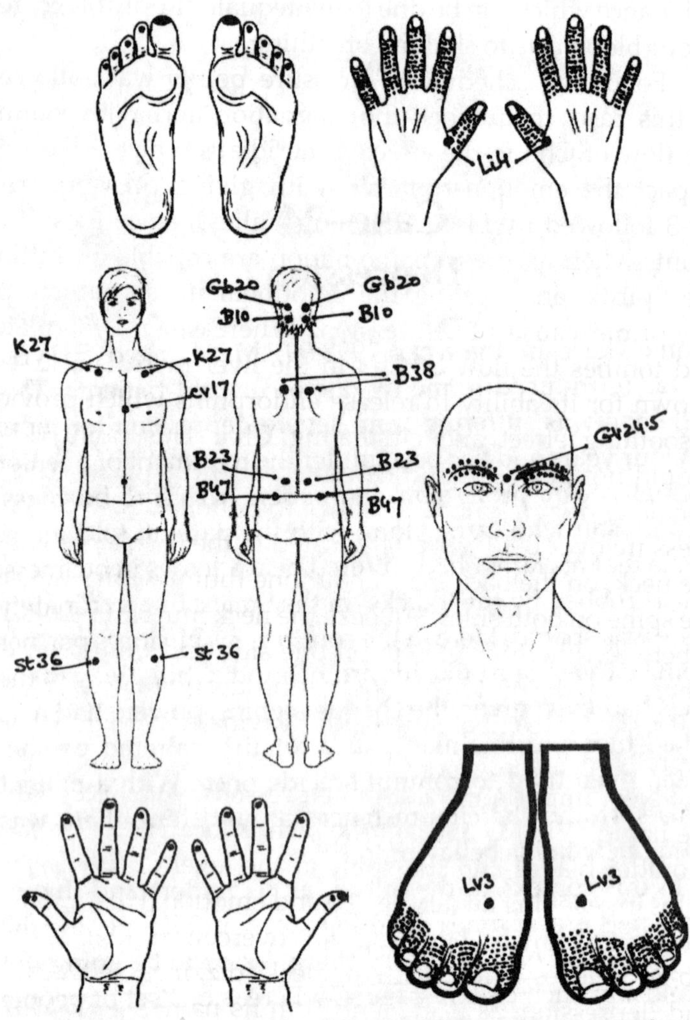

a pretty long time without letting it out or expressing the same, it ends up into 'depression' by turning the inward anger against yourself. It could thus be repressed emotions or 'Stagnant' energy. The flow of Ch'i in the liver meridian. It could also be caused by the deficiency of Vitamins 'C' and 'E', which can be made good by the use of salad of parsley and cucumber, dressed with fresh lemon juice. Deep breathing is also considered useful in overcoming emotional imbalance which can be due to inadequate supply of oxygen in our blood due to shallow breathing.

Following schedule of pressure points was followed in this case, to unblock the stagnation and rejuvenating the flow of Ch'i in the effected meridians which adversely impact the emotions. Started with giving pressure over Lv-3 followed by Li-4 (Adjoining Valley), since these two points when used as a combination are capable of 'Lifting the Spirits' and healing the emotional upsets which are the prime cause of depression. Whereas, Lv-3 regulates and tonifies the flow of Ch'i in the liver meridian, Li-4 is known for its ability to release endorphins which provide a soothing effect and circulating Ch'i. This point (Li-4) should not be pressed in case the patient happens to be a female and is pregnant. This has to be followed by giving pressure over B-10, which is located in the upper portion of the neck, on the back side, about one thumb width outside the spine on both sides. Squeeze the neck muscle by holding it between the four fingers on one side and thumb on the other, from the back. This point is the key point to overcome stiffness, and combat stress and heaviness in the head and depression.

Next important point to be pressed is B-38, known by the name, 'Vital Diaphragm' which is located between the shoulder blades and the spine at the level of the heart. It helps in relieving anxiety, grief, and emotional disturbances and is extremely beneficial in overcoming depression. Gb-20 relieves headache, stiff neck, dizziness, irritability, and depression, as is evident from its name, i.e. 'Gates of Consciousness', its location is shown in the figure. It as been found to be highly beneficial in overcoming depression. K-27, which is located in the hollow below the collarbone next to the breast bone, also helps overcome anxiety and depression. Follow this by pressing Gv-24.5, which is located between the eyebrows, as shown in figure. This tones up the endocrine system, particularly the pituitary gland, tones up the entire body, overcomes head congestion as also emotional disturbances and depression. Yet another important point to be pressed is Cv-17 (Sea of Tranquility), which is located in the centre of the breast bone. It as been found to be of immense importance in relieving nervousness, grief, depression, hysteria and other emotional disturbances.

B-23, located in the middle of the waist, half way between the rib cage and the hip bone on the inner edge, relieves depression, fear, and trauma. B-47 reduces, muscle tension, depression, and fear, to the followed by pressing St-36(Three Mile Point), a point known to tone up muscles of the entire body, balance emotions and thus help in overcoming depression. Pressure can be given for 30 to 60 seconds. As has been mentioned earlier too, during the first three to four sessions, pressure can be given over all the pressure points discussed above and thereafter, some points can be pressed during one session and the rest of the points can be pressed next time and so on to get the results. Giving pressure over the thumbs, big toes and over the skin (upper part) of the fingers, shown by the dots in the figure with the help of a spring ring, which is easily available in the market as also giving pressure over the eyebrows as shown in the figure also helps a lot in overcoming depression.

While handling patients of depression always try to co-manage them with conventional medicine. Close coordination between the psychiatrist and the therapist is of prime importance. Whereas, in chronic cases, the patient has been getting medication and the psychiatrist has no other option but to resort to using sedatives. As such the patient is seldom able to come to his/her true self. It becomes difficult to make out in case the therapy being given to overcome emotional as well as physical stress, as also to overcome chemical imbalances in the system is showing any positive effect. This is possible, only when some of the medication is partially withdrawn or the medication is slowly withdrawn by tapering. But this should be done strictly in consultation with the consent of the attending physician. In the instant case, fortunately, the psychiatrist attending Mr. J himself was a believer of Naturopathy and was an open-minded doctor and there was no problem in regulating the medicine.

The patient was kept just on maintenance dose after around 20 sessions or so. As a result thereof, the patient responded well to the treatment. In all around 27-28 sessions were given and during every session, patient's counseling was also done to get best of the results. By the time his treatment was stopped, he had resumed his work. While stopping the treatment, his son, who used to take keen interest in his father's recovery, was trained to give him the therapy once or twice a week for a few months more to stabilize the results.

□

Case–25
Belching

In the year 2002, I happened to treat a 54 yrs old female Mrs. G, wife of an Air Marshal in the Indian Airforce. She was suffering from severe gastric problem and the peculiar feature in her case was that she used to 'Belch' at such a high pitch that it was not only a cause of embarrassment to her but also a major irritant to the people around. Surprisingly, her belching used to commence at the slightest pressure over any part of her body, i.e. even in case her hand was held and pressed a bit. She confided in me and told that, whenever she has to go with her husband in the parties as a protocol, she is surrounded by the wives of her husbands' juniors and she felt scared for the reason that some lady will come and hug her or hold her hand firmly just to say, madam you are looking so good, etc... and that she would start belching, thereby creating a scene. She further told that she had tried almost every possible antacid and has been observing all the prescribed food restrictions, but nothing has helped her in overcoming the problem of belching loudly.

In this context, needless to say, many people suffer from this sort of a problem and different people have different symptoms/intensity, e.g. gas formation, belching, flatulence, burning sensation in the region of esophagus, etc. One can easily conclude that faulty diet could be the prime cause. Some people could be sensitive to a particular type of food or the other, hot and spicy meals, fried/fast food, etc. Stress could be another underlying factor responsible for

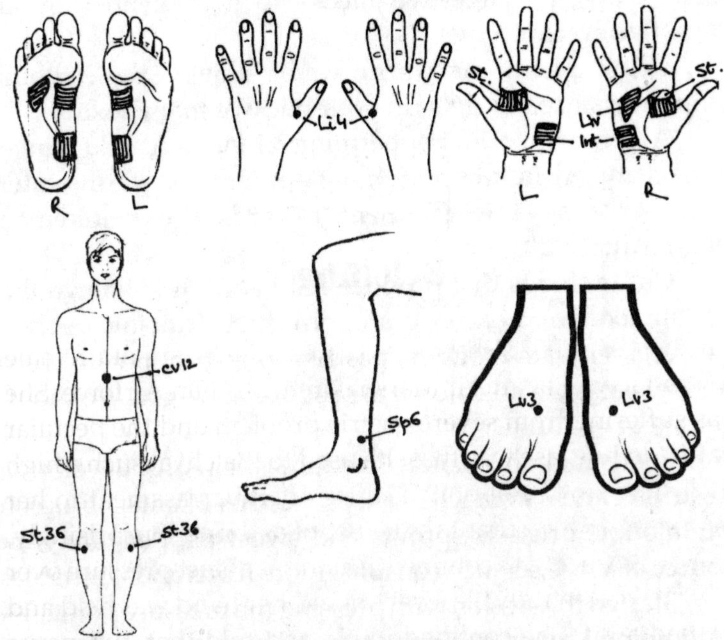

the aggravation of this condition. Several other conditions that promote excessive flatulence/belching/bloating could also be due to peptic ulcers, stomach infections, gall stones, IBS (a blend of stomach pain, gas formation, bloating and irregular bowl movements), lactose intolerance (i.e. inability to digest milk or milk products) as well as certain food allergies. Swallowing too much air while chewing can also make you pass more gas. Instead of resorting to antacids, our goal should be to correct our lifestyle and dietary plan to suit our body requirement by taking help of some good dietician. Besides, resorting to acupressure treatment as per treatment plan discussed below, gave certain 'tips' to the patient that helped her and the same are being listed out here.

Eat small meals (eat like a bird) — doing so helps reduce the amount of bacteria in the stomach, thereby creating less gas. This also leads to the stomach producing lesser amount of digestive juices which are gentler on our digestive system.

Drink plenty of warm water slowly but without stopping, since this gets rid your body of many toxins.

A few drops of peppermint, cinnamon, and ginger extract mixed in a cup of water (preferably warm water) may serve as a replacement towards the requirement of an 'Antacid'.

Cut on foods that produce flatulence. It is known that certain foods, e.g. bacon, bran, corn chips, fruit juice, gelatin desserts, graham crackers, pastries, popcorn, potato chips, and wheat germ are known to produce more gas. We should try to cut on these.

Foods high in Vitamin C reduces the risk of developing gastritis and stomach cancer. Citrus fruits, broccoli, cantaloupe, brussels sprouts and sweet peppers are good source of Vit. C, as such consume more fruits and vegetables.

Started the session with pressing the pressure point Li-4, 'Adjoining Valley', the point which lies in the web between the thumb and the index finger. It improves the intestinal activity besides relieving abdominal distention and also constipation that leads to the formation of gas. Next, I gave pressure over St-36 (Three Mile Point) as shown in the figure. This point also relieves indigestion, prevents gas formation and bloating. Moderate yet firm pressure needs to be given over this point. You will find that most of the time I have followed point Sp-6, 'Three Meeting Point' immediately after pressing St.-36. The reason behind is that by doing so the effectiveness of both these points multiplies manifolds. As such make it a point that pressure over this combination has to be given in conjunction to drive maximum benefit out of them. However, make sure that pressure over Sp-6 is not given to pregnant women.

Finally gave pressure over Lv-3, as shown in figure to overcome stress and thereby get relief from distention, nausea, vomiting, and abdominal pain too that is, at times, caused due to distention. Followed by giving pressure over Cv-12, as shown to overcome indigestion, heartburn, abdominal pain, and constipation.

Also give pressure over the reflex areas pertaining to the main digestive organs, as depicted in figure at the end of the book, e.g. liver, stomach, intestines (large/small), etc., of our digestive system to stimulate them for better digestion. The patient responded to the treatment well and by the time six to seven sessions were over, the incidence of belching reduced by around 35-40%, thereafter she was asked to come thrice a week only for subsequent sessions. In all around 18 sessions were given. At the end of the last session, a chart indicating the pressure points to be pressed once a week (as self help) was handed over to her, so that she can herself keep her system in perfect condition.

□

Case–26
Hiccups

I recall the case of an old gentleman Mr. B, aged around 67 yrs. who was brought to me in the year 2008 for management of 'Hiccups'. The patient informed me that his problem started about four years ago but at that time, he used to get hiccups only once in a while and the problem used to get resolved by taking luke warm water or simply by diverting attention. But slowly the duration as well as the intensity of the hiccups has increased. He added that for the past week or so, he is not able to recall if the hiccups have stopped even for a while and that his sleep is also getting disturbed due to this problem.

In this regard, let us admit that despite all the advances medical science has made over the years, science could not find a sure cure for this sort of annoying spasm. A hiccup is an audible tic, the phrenic nerve that excites the muscles of the diaphragm, results into uncontrollable spasms. At times some food stuck in our esophagus also triggers a nerve spasm in the esophagus where it meets the stomach. So far as the hiccups come and vanish on their own, there is no cause for alarm, however, when they persist for long, it could be an indication of a more serious problem. Generally, people recovering from surgery get hiccups or it may be attributed to body's reaction to anesthesia. But prolonged/recurrent hiccups may give an indication of some developing kidney problem or an abscess or a tumor in the chest or esophagus. Also, some people might develop

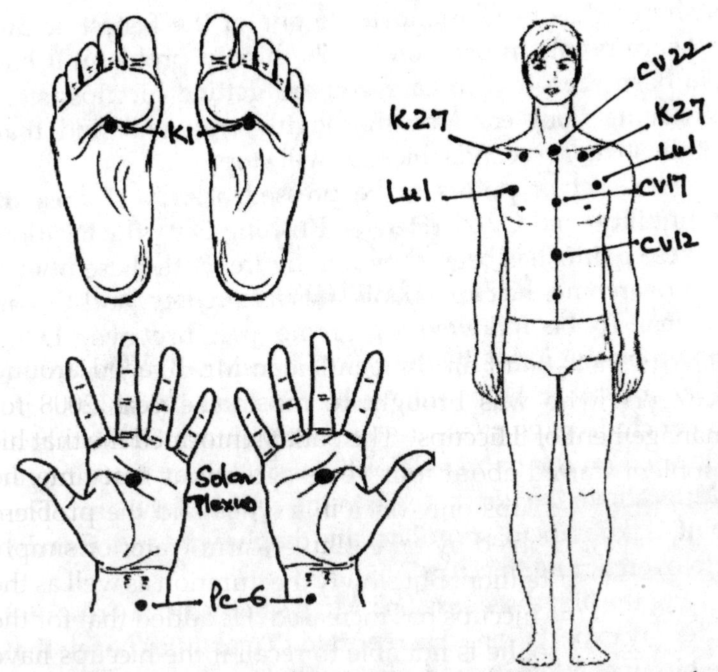

hiccups due to some psychological reasons, e.g. due to fear. The more you try to suppress it or you get tense, the more it aggravates. Generally, sitting in a relaxed position and sipping luke warm water solves the problem.

The following schedule of pressure points proved beneficial in the case of Mr. B. Started giving pressure over K-1 point as shown in the figure, this point is also called the 'Solar Plexus Point'. Unless hiccup is due to some deep-seated cause, giving pressure over just this point is sufficient to overcome the problem. Followed by giving pressure over Cv-12, which is located almost midway between the bottom of the breast bone and the naval. In case pressure over this point is given when the patient is empty stomach, it yields even better results. It relieves hiccups, emotional stress. K-27, which is located just below the collar bone, as shown, tonifies the kidneys, and is considered key detoxification point. It helps overcome hiccups, chest congestion and anxiety. Tw-17, which is located just below the Earlobe, as shown, has been found to be one of the fastest acting pressure points in overcoming the hiccup problem. It has also been seen that in case you are getting hiccups, start massaging your ear lobe thoroughly, you will find that within 30 to 60 seconds, hiccups will stop.

Next set of points to be pressed are Cv-17 (Sea of Tranquility) and Cv-22 (Heaven Rushing Out), the location of these points has been shown in figure. Both these points help overcome, hiccups, panic attacks, anxiety, and throat spasms. To be followed by giving pressure over Lu-1, known by the name 'Letting Go', is found near the crease of the armpit, it helps relieve hiccups and breathlessness. To conclude gave pressure over Pc-6 (Inner Gate), which is located on the palm side of the wrist, about three finger widths above the wrist crease in the centre of the arm. This point is known to stimulate the diaphragm and thereby help overcoming 'hiccups'.

For the first three sessions, Mr. B's body did not respond as per my expectations. He reported that at times he felt that the hiccups' intensity had reduced but soon he was back to square one. But when he came for the fourth session, he had some thing positive to report. He informed that previous night he was able to sleep for four hours peacefully after around 10 days or so. He admitted that now he has some hope that he will recover soon. In all 13 sessions proved enough. Stopped his treatment with instructions that in case of recurrence he should inform me without loss of time, so that corrective measures can be taken. But fortunately he had no problem for more than six months. One day after about eight months or so, he called to take appointment saying he had hiccup for about a minute or two but it stopped on its own. I told him there was no need to panic and he can give massage like pressure on his ear lobes as and when he gets hiccups. Told him to come, in case it recurs for long or frequently. But fortunately he did not have to come for treatment again.

□

Case–27
U.T.I.

In the year 2001, a doctor patient of mine (herself a medical practitioner in conventional medicine), who had taken treatment of her prolapsed disc from me about three years ago, phoned me that one of her colleagues aged 27 yrs, who is working in her hospital has been time and again suffering from UTI problem. She wanted to know if there is any cure in acupressure for this problem too. I told her that she can bring the patient in the evening of the weekend. Dr. (Mrs.) A, informed that she has been having this problem from the age of 20 yrs or so and every time she suffers, she takes a course of antibiotics and within four to six months again the problem crops up. She also complained of incontinence after her first delivery about two years back.

Whereas, the kidneys, bladder and urethra are the main components of the urinary tract, bladder infection is caused frequently for the reason that urine stays in the urinary bladder/tract for a longer duration and that a cause good enough for the bacteria to have more time to infect and multiply. Whereas the incidence of UTI in female is very common (even in little girls) for the reason that the size of the urethra is much shorter in women than in men, but men over 50 years do suffer from urinary infection because of enlarged prostate. The problem also crops up by an infection of the mucus membranes of the bladder by bacteria that moves in from the intestines or the anus. The symptoms are frequent urination, less quantity, burning

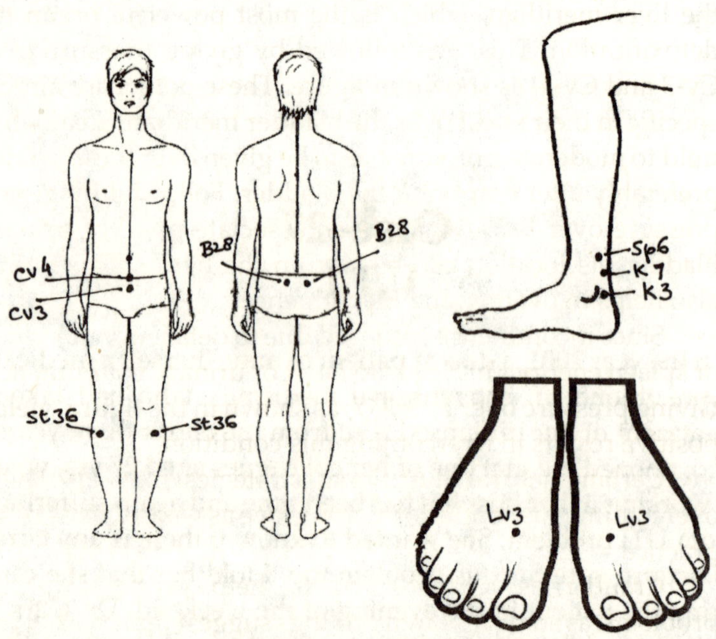

and painful sensation while passing urine. At times the condition may be accompanied with fever too. Incidence of bladder infections is more in the patients who do not take enough fluids. Drink 8 to 10 glasses of water every day.

Following schedule of pressure points was followed to overcome both urinary tract infection and incontinence. Pressed St-36 and Sp-6 (Three Yin Meeting) points as have been shown in the figure. Whereas, St-36, tones up the muscles of the entire body, it becomes even more potent and revitalizes the entire body when pressed along with Sp-6, which further tonifies three meridians at the same time, i.e. kidney, liver and spleen. This point is known for its stimulating effect over these three meridians and for being helpful in overcoming any sort of female problem. But pressure over this point should not be given to pregnant women. Next point pressed was Lv-3 that lies between the big toe and the second toe, as shown in the figure. This point tonifies the liver and regulates the flow of Ch'i in the liver meridian, which is the most powerful organ for detoxification. This was followed by giving pressure over Cv-3 and Cv-4, as shown in figure. These points are almost specific in their effect over the bladder meridian. Steady but mild to moderate pressure has to be given over these points, preferably after emptying the bladder. Followed by giving pressure over B-28, which is an associate point of urinary bladder, its location can be seen in the figure. This points also helps in overcoming incontinence.

Since incontinence is caused due to deficiency in kidney or spleen energy, this leads to bowl or urinary incontinence. Giving pressure over K-3; K-7, as shown in the figure, yields positive results in overcoming this condition.

Certain natural nutritional strategies may also help overcoming this condition as a curative as well as preventive practice.

Cranberries are believed to help prevent urinary problems, as some research findings suggest that cranberries slow the growth of bacteria by making urine more acidic. Other studies show that cranberries keep bacteria from clinging to your urinary tract. The bacteria slip right throughout of your body. As such drink cranberry juice regularly in case you have a tendency to suffer from UTI very frequently.

Drink lots of water, at least 8 to 10 glasses every day as water can wash away the bacteria from our body. Pale yellow color of urine indicates that you need more water. Take Vit. C, at least 500 mg/day, as this will make your urine more acidic, making it difficult for the bacteria to grow.

By the time six sessions were given, the patient reported substantial recovery. In all 11-12 sessions did the job. The patient and the doctor who had brought this patient, later on informed me that they have also learnt these pressure points and they have given pressure to the female coming to them with this condition and many of them got benefited. □

Case–28
Bed Wetting

About eight years ago, a five-year-old child was brought to my clinic who suffered from bed wetting problem. His mother told me that earlier up to the age of three years or so, the child never had this sort of a problem and she told that the previous night the child was beaten by his father and that this problem of the child was becoming a cause of tension between them. I told his father that there is nothing new with their child as almost all children wet the bed some time or the other. They do not do so willingly, rather they too feel humiliated. As such the child should be tutored to be more careful while sleeping, pass urine before going to bed. Parents should wake them up in case they notice a particular trend that after going to bed, the child passes urine after two, three or four hours. Told them that beating the child will induce a sense of fear in the child that would further aggravate the condition. Further, proving brought out to light that incidence of bed wetting were there in the family in their yester years too. Because, it is a known thing that heredity factor plays a significant role in this sort of a condition, we forget our past easily. Boys wet the bed more than the girls.

Causes of bed wetting include, lack of training, excessive intake of fluids, anxiety and fear, mental deficiency, epilepsy, meningomyocele, pyelonephritis, epispadias, phimosis, and thread worm infestation, etc. It may also be owing to the deficiency in water element, which means kidney and

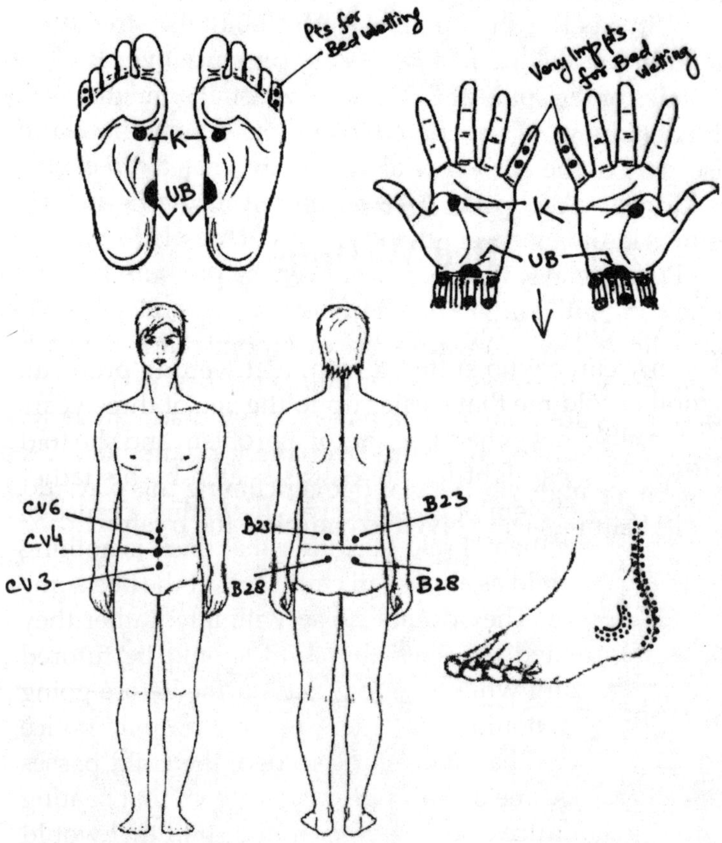

urinary bladder meridians need to be strengthened. U.T.I. may also be the cause behind and once U.T.I. is cured, bed wetting also stops on its own. Severe respiratory restrictions like sleep apnea can also cause bed wetting.

Acupressure treatment has been found to be very effective in overcoming this problem. Gave pressure over Cv-3 (Zhongji), Cv-4, (Guan Yuan), and Cv-6 (Sea of Ch'i), the exact location of these points has been shown in figure. Cv-3 lies at the centre along the midline of the abdomen, slightly above the pubic bone. It is known for its ability to treat disorders of urinary tract. Cv-4 lies a little above Cv-3.

It stimulates the kidneys. Cv-6 is located a little above Cv-4 and a little below the umbilicus. This point too strengthens the kidneys. Follow this by giving pressure over B-23, on the sides of the spine at the level of waist. It strengthens the Ch'i of kidneys, is considered to be a major point in treating disorders of the euro-genital system and has a direct effect on kidneys. Also press B-28 as shown in the figure. This point is known to strengthen the Ch'i of the bladder.

Pressure may also be given over the pressure points as indicated on the little fingers of both hands and soles. This was followed by giving pressure over point marked over the wrist. Also give pressure over points marked in the figure. These pressure points pertains to kidney meridian as well as genitals. Giving pressure over these points have been found to be highly beneficial in over coming this condition. In all 11 sittings were given to complete the treatment.

□

Case–29
Cramps in Calf

I recall having attended a patient, 55 yrs. old female, who was admitted in a famous hospital of New Delhi, in the year 1995. The female Mrs. S was admitted there with multiple problems and was admitted in a room that was just adjacent to the room, where my mother who had fractured her hip bone (neck of femur) was also admitted. This female used to get 'cramps' in her calf muscle very frequently and used to cry at the top of her voice. It had almost become a practice that the moment she used to cry, I would rush out of my mother's room to pacify her. Frankly speaking, I had assumed the self-acclaimed role of treating her by giving her relief from the pain and agony she used to get by the cramp, so that my mother is not disturbed. Subsequently, I found that the attendant(s) of that patient, started rushing towards our room, the moment their patient got the cramp, when they noticed that by holding certain points for a few moments she gets relief and stops crying.

As a matter of fact, cramps can develop anywhere in the body, however, generally they occur in the muscle(s) that have been over used (generally caused due to muscular tension). During a cramp, the nerves of the affected muscle become 'hyperactive' and causes extreme contraction of the involved muscle, resulting into excruciating pain in the affected area and the patient is forced to cry with pain. At times, even if you slightly stretch your legs, cramps occur. Dehydration may be yet another causative factor at the back

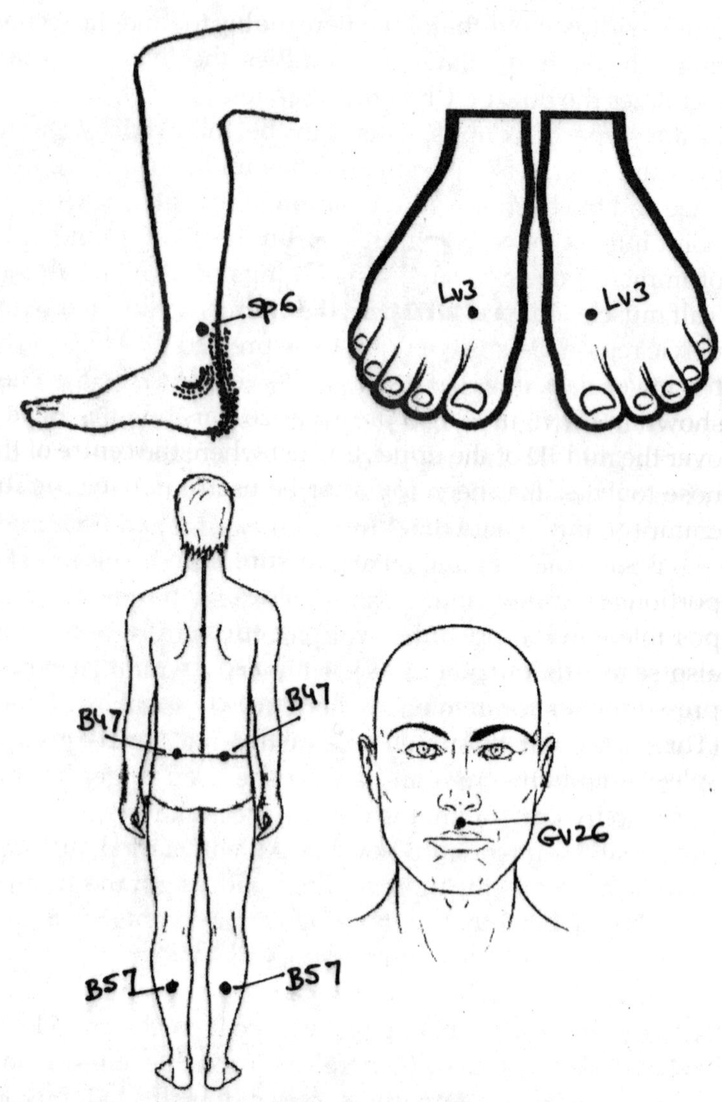

of this condition. Pressing certain pressure points provide immense spontaneous relief to the patient suffering from cramps. The points to be pressed are:

Lv-3 point is perhaps the point, importance of which cannot be overemphasized. It lies on the top of the foot, two finger widths above the joint where the big toe and the second finger meet. It regulates and tonifies the liver meridian, facilitates the flow of 'Ch'i and is capable of providing relief in any type of cramps. This may be followed by giving pressure over B-57, a point that lies midway between the knee and the heel, just at the bottom of the calf muscle. This point hurts a lot on being pressed but has been found to be of immense use in overcoming cramps particularly that of 'calf muscle'. In case, however, the cramps are located in the pelvic region, B-47 is the point to be pressed. It is located on the lower back between L-2 and L-3 vertebrae, as has been shown in the figure. Also press Gv-26, this point is located over the middle of the upper lip, just where the centre of the nose touches. Has been found to be useful in over coming cramps, fainting, and dizziness.

Besides above, also give pressure around the shaded portion over the ankles, both sides, over both feet if possible. Giving pressure over the effected foot only will also serve the purpose. Last of all also give massage like pressure over the achilles tendon area covering Sp-6 point (Three Meeting Point) that stimulates kidney, liver, and spleen simultaneously.

□

Case–30
Sea Sickness

It was somewhere in the year 1999, I was travelling to 'Havelock Islands' from Port Blair in a steamer, on a trip. Sitting next to me was a couple, a diamond merchant by profession, who was travelling along-with his wife, perhaps on a honeymoon trip. Barely an hours journey was completed, when all of a sudden, the female in her late twenties developed severe 'Sea Sickness'. The severity of the sickness was so high that she could not sit on her seat barely even for one or two minutes and had to rush to the basin, on the deck to vomit. She was belching too at a very high pitch, disturbing co-passenger and every one on the deck were feeling scary since sea sickness spreads like a viral infection, i.e. at the sight of some one vomiting, others too start vomiting.

I kept waiting for around 4-5 minutes and finally when his wife went to vomit, I told her husband, who was sitting next to me, to press K-1 point in her palms and soles, when she comes back. That young man had perhaps heard about 'acupressure', and requested me to help in case I could. When the female came back, they exchanged seats and I started giving her pressure over K-1 point, also known by the name 'Bubbling Springs'. In the first go, I could barely give her pressure over the point for 10-15 seconds, on her both palms that she had to rush back for vomiting. But by the time she came back in a minute or so, pressure had shown its effect. I again commenced giving pressure. After

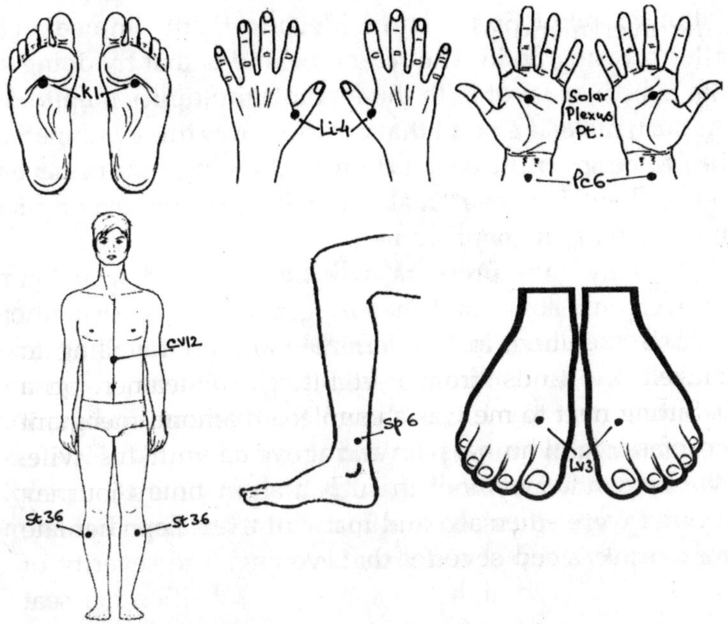

giving pressure over both the palms on K-1 point, I started giving her pressure over the same point in her soles too. Having given pressure for about one minute over all the four limbs on this point, I found that she had stabilized a bit.

Thereafter, I started pressing the pressure point Pc-6, this point is known by the name 'Inner Gate' and is located about three finger widths above the wrist crease in the middle, as shown in figure. It is known to relieve vomiting in Sea Voyagers. This point is so potent that it is capable of controlling vomiting during pregnancy as well as the side effect of chemotherapy. Next point pressed was Li-4, 'Adjoining Valley', the point which lies in the web between the thumb and the index finger. It improves the intestinal activity besides relieving abdominal distention and also constipation that leads to the formation of gas. Next, I gave pressure over St.-36 (Three Mile Point) as shown in the figure. This point also relieves indigestion, prevents gas formation and bloating. Moderate yet firm pressure needs to be given over this point. You will find that most of the time I have followed point Sp-6, 'Three Meeting Point' immediately after pressing St-36. The reason behind is that by doing so the effectiveness of both these points multiplies manifolds. As such make it a point that pressure over this combination has to be given in conjunction to drive maximum benefit out of them. However, make sure that pressure over Sp-6 is not given to pregnant women.

Finally gave pressure over Lv-3, as shown in figure to overcome stress and thereby get relief from distention, nausea, vomiting, and abdominal pain too that is at times caused due to continuous vomiting. Followed by giving pressure over Cv-12, as shown to overcome indigestion, heartburn, abdominal pain and above all the 'Sea Sickness'. She responded so well in such a short time that people around were surprised and many of them approached me for a drink/a cup of coffee that evening.

□

Case–31
Hot Flashes

In this case, I am not quoting any specific case history but this topic is being included for the reason that so far we have handled hundreds of female in the age group of 40 to 52 yrs, who come with 'Hot flashes' problem. It has been observed that whereas a good number of female attain menopause without facing much discomfort, but those are a lucky few. As a matter of fact, hot flushes are body's reaction to the decreased supply of the hormone, 'estrogen' which occurs in due course as women attain the age of menopause. In those cases where the downfall in the production of estrogen is gradual, not much discomfort is felt by the female. But in the case(s) where the production of estrogen is abruptly stopped by the ovaries, the women have a real tough time. Most of the times, they occur at night and at times are followed one after the other, resulting into hot and sweaty restless/sleepless nights. At times, the sufferer feels flames coming out from her body and tends to throw away as many clothes as possible while immediately thereafter, she may feel chilled and try to pull on even 2-3 blankets at a time. Certain female, during this transition period of menopause also experience terrible mood swings.

Menopause, i.e. cessation of monthly cycle signals the end of a women's fertile period, and she attains freedom from those painful periods, hassle of adopting birth control measures and fear of getting pregnant. In case a woman does not get periods for six months consecutively, it marks

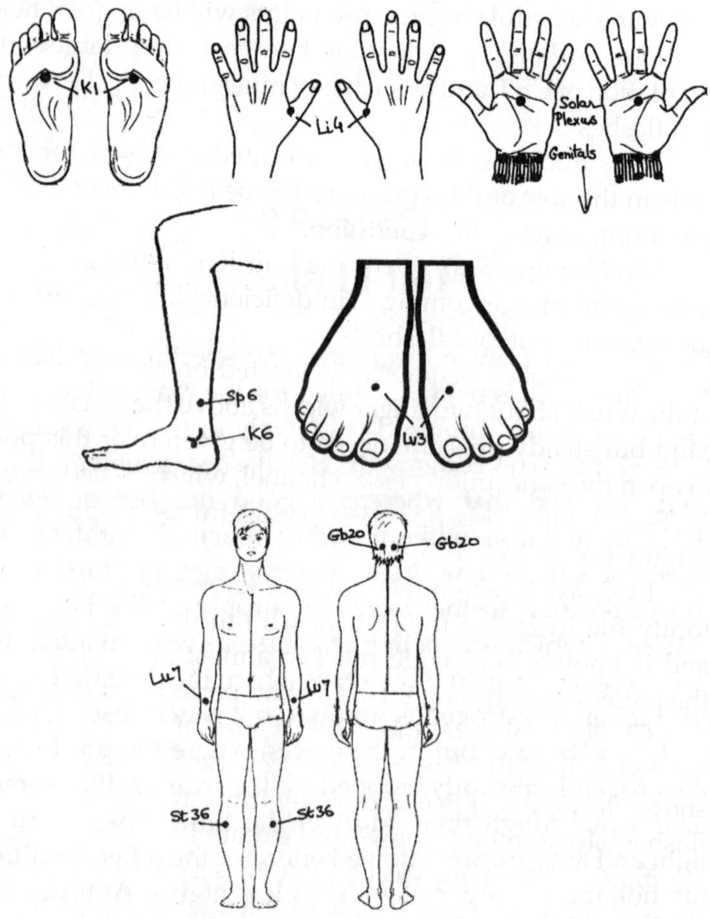

the beginning of the menopause cycle. But to avoid the risk of getting pregnant, she should adopt family planning measures, till at least one full year period passes without menstruation. Other symptoms besides hot flushes include, vaginal dryness, depression besides mood swings and hot flushes. This happens because of 'Yin' deficiency that leads to lack of internal cooling ability in the body. As such the best natural way to overcome this condition is to stimulate those pressure points which nourish the 'Yin' deficiency and in establishing a good 'Yin-Yang' balance in the body.

Following schedule of pressure points will be of great help:

Li-4, 'Adjoining Valley', is known to re-establish the circulation of Ch'i, and as such is of much relief in alleviating 'hot flashes'.

K-1, 'Bubbling Springs', is located between the two pads in the sole and is considered to be highly beneficial in providing relief in this condition.

K-6 (Shining Sea), opens the 'Yin-Ren' meridian and is thus useful in overcoming 'Yin deficiency', thus removing the root cause of 'hot flashes'.

Lu-7, (Broken Sequence) is located on the thumb side of the wrist, about two finger widths above the wrist crease. Mild but steady pressure needs to be given over this point to open the conception vessel channel, which is also known as 'Sea of Yin'. This point is very useful when pressed in conjunction with K-6.

Lv-3, as shown in the figure, is known to regulate and tonify the liver and the flow of Ch'i in the liver meridian and is known to provide relief in almost all symptoms to the patient undergoing the transition period of menopause.

Gb-20, known by the name, 'Gates of Consciousness', located below the base of skull, in the hollow space, as shown in figure. It is extremely helpful in overcoming hot flashes, stress, mood swings and irritability.

Sp-6, 'Three Ying Meeting Point', is a crucial point to be pressed for almost any female problem(s) as it strengthens the 'Yin' of three meridians, viz. kidneys, liver, and spleen at the same time. Helps stimulate Ch'i in the entire body and circulation of blood too.

To finish the session, give pressure over St-36, as in the figure, to tone up the whole body, muscles and getting much sought after relief from 'hot flushes'.

Besides following the pressure point regime, the patient was advised to increase their consumption of 'Soya' products, e.g. tofu and other products containing more of 'Soy'. This need to be done based on a research study conducted by American, Finnish, and Japanese researchers that singles out soy products as a possible treatment for menopausal symptoms. In yet another study it was found that only 9 to 10% Japanese women suffer from menopausal symptoms as compared to over 50% women who reported menopausal symptoms in Western European countries. This was attributed to the factor that Japanese women consume more of 'Soy' than Western women do. It said Soy foods contain a natural estrogenic compound that may serve as a hot flash reliever.

Since caffeine tends to raise the blood pressure and the heart rate slightly, it is better to cut on coffee consumption to reduce the incidence of 'hot flashes'.

Going the 'Yogic' way, a recent study has revealed that women given the training in "Slow, Deep-Breathing Exercises" were able to reduce their hot flashes by as good as 50%. As such the patients coming for acupressure treatment to overcome 'hot flashes' were also advised to get in touch with a Yoga expert to teach them appropriate disease specific breathing relaxation techniques, which shall bring much sought after relief from the amount of discomfort they experience due to hot flashes.

□

Case–32
Writer's Cramps

A case of 'writer's cramps' was brought to me in the year 1999. The patient was a 16-year-old boy who had this problem and was supposed to write Board examination that year. His mother, who came with him, told me that she has seen a good number of doctors and almost all of them have told her, after conducting lots of tests and giving medicines, that perhaps the boy shall have to take help of typewriters/ computers, his entire life since he used to get severe cramps in his hand the moment he wrote even 5-6 sentences at a stretch.

This condition is an occupationally induced dystonia. Attempt to write is inhibited by dystonic posturing of hand and arm and the person is not able to write. In other words, the hand can be used for any other purpose except writing. Perhaps, no drugs have been proved to be effective. The probable contributory factors could be sustained muscular contractions and electrolyte imbalance.

Pressing the following pressure points provided immense relief to the patient suffering from Writer's Cramps. The points pressed were:

Lv-3 point is perhaps the point, importance of which cannot be overemphasized. It lies on the top of the foot, two finger widths above the joint where the big toe and the second finger meet. It regulates and tonifies the liver meridian, facilitates the flow of Ch'i and is capable of

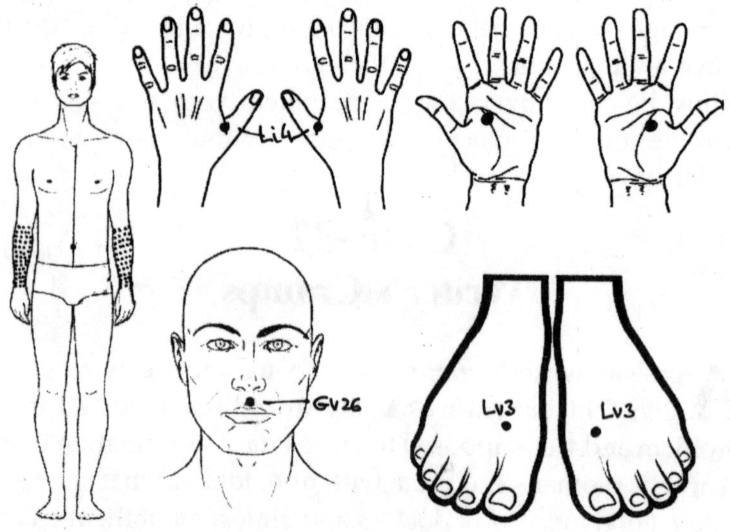

providing relief in any type of cramps. Also press Gv-26, this point is located over the middle of the upper lip, just where the centre of the nose touches. Has been found to be useful in over coming cramps, fainting, and dizziness.

Besides the aforesaid pressure points, also press at the point that falls where the middle finger touches your palm, when the fist is closed. This point has been found to be highly beneficial in over coming writer's cramps. Pressure has to be given only over the effected hand. Also gave pressure at Li-4 ('Adjoining Valley'), this is known for its ability to relieve any sort of pain in the body, as on pressing this point our body releases endorphins, the natural pain killers as also it helps restore the flow of Ch'i through the body. It also helps into elimination of toxins through bowels, removes stagnation of Ch'i too. Pregnant women should not be given pressure over this point.

The boy responded so well to the treatment that within eight sessions, he was able to write without much discomfort. As a precaution, I asked him to tie loose crape bandage over his hand while writing for a few days. Also gave another four sessions thereafter, every alternate day. Thus, he could over come his problem within 12 sessions and he could write his board exams, without any problem whatsoever.

□

Case–33
Low Back Pain/Cervical

Somewhere in the year 2000, an officer from the Civil Services, Mr. G, aged about 50 yrs. was brought to my clinic with severe low back ache as also cervical spondylosis. He told me that he has taken every possible treatment including physiotherapy, he gets relief for some time but soon the pain returns and he is back to square one. Further, he told me that after almost half an hour of work, he has to lie down on bed even in his office, which he had got in the side room of his chamber (since he was a pretty senior officer, he could have that facility). He further shared that the pain used to aggravate in case he sat even for 30 minutes at a stretch on his chair, despite he has got a very comfortable cushion on his office chair. He told that while taking a meeting, he deliberately keeps his water tumbler in the other corner on a table since he cannot afford to sit for long and under the disguise to get water he gets up from his chair, walks all the way to the corner to take water. In other words, he communicated that the pain becomes intolerable by sitting for even half an hour and gets better by some movement.

In this context, it may be understood that episodic low back pain is due to rupture of anular ligament. There is extrusion of soft tissue material from nuclear pulpous. As we age, the water content of the disc decreases. Spondylosis between L-5-S-1 results in pain radiating down the back of thigh, outer side of the lower leg and outer side of the foot to

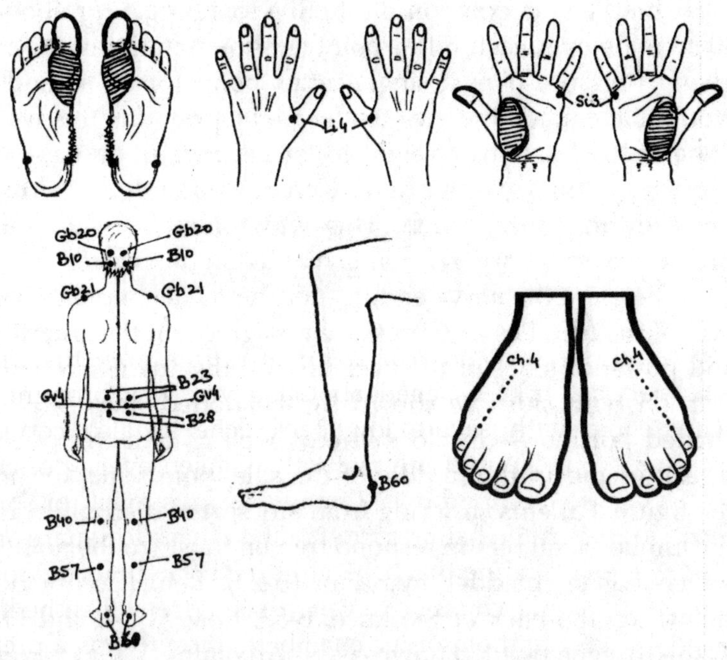

the fifth toe. Whereas, in case of lesion between L-2 and L-3 pain radiates down the front of thigh. Disc prolapsed pain is aggravated by sitting, lifting and coughing, sneezing, laughing and straining to defecate. Whereas, cervical spondylosis is a degenerative condition of cervical vertebra and may be symptomless or cause neurological symptoms. Clinical manifestations are the patients with clumsy numb hands, at times the pain radiating from the region of the chest to the arm producing a feel like that of 'angina' pain. This condition is primarily caused because of faulty posture. Working on computers for long hours, watching TV sitting or lying in a wrong posture, driving long distances sitting in uncomfortable/wrong posture could be the other underlying causes for the onset of this problem.

I started his treatment with the following action plan: Began with stimulating the lumbo sacral region over the soles and the palms. Direct pressure was given on the areas marked 'xxxxxx' on the lumbo-sacral part for about 30 seconds over each reflex point as shown in figure, since giving pressure over a single reflex point for 30 seconds would have made the area tender to the pressure, this was done in the fractions of eight to ten seconds in one go on every point thus giving pressure on one point three to four times during one session. This was followed by giving pressure over the trigger points marked in the figure.

These are the nerve endings for the sciatic nerve in the heel of the feet. Besides, pressure was given on the anterior and posterior sides of the heel, around the ankles on both feet, on both sides as shown by the dotted lines — the shaded portion — in clockwise as well as anti-clockwise direction and in the middle of the sole, points marked in the figure. Patients suffering from any sort of discomfort in the lumbo sacral region respond tremendously to the points which fall on bladder meridian (B-23), B-40 (Command point)- on the back of the knee, B-57, B-60, GV-4, and Li-4, this trigger point (known as — Adjoining Valley) over the large intestine meridian gives relief to pain in any part of the body by helping in circulating the Ch'i in the entire body. The precise location of these points has been shown in the figure.

After giving pressure over the reflex points discussed above, pressure was given over Gb-20, which is located in the hollow below the base of the skull to over come stiffness in the neck and upper back pain. Followed by pressure over Gb-21, 'Shoulder Well' which lies midway between the neck and the outer edge of shoulder. This point is by and large very tender and has to be pressed very gently, simultaneously over both sides of the shoulder, the patient may be advised to take slow but deep breaths to get maximum benefit. This point restores normal flow of Ch'i in the lungs. This point should not be pressed in case of female patients, who are carrying. Next apply pressure over B-10, 'Heavenly Pillars', it is located about one and a half inches below the base of the skull, two finger widths on both side of the spine simultaneously. Relieves, headache, exhaustion, stiffness in the shoulders, and swollen eyes. Si-3 is yet another point to be pressed to overcome stiffness in the shoulder region, as has been shown in the figure. Press this point firmly with moderate pressure, for about a minute.

Also work over the reflex areas of the cervical vertebrae on the big toes and the thumbs, as shown in the figure, i.e. up to the first knuckle of the thumbs and the entire big toe on both hands and feet. Also work over the pads below the big toe and thumbs in the palms, this area reflects the scapula blades and provides lot of relief to the patients suffering from cervical problem.

Within three sessions, Mr. G, reported that he has been having a feeling of wellness and by the time 5-6 sessions were completed, he reported 30-35% relief. After that he was asked to come every alternate day, so as to prolong his span of treatment without increasing the number of sessions. In all 14 sessions did the job. He brought his wife also for her cervical treatment and she was also benefitted. Informed me that he has stopped using the bed in his office, now he could sit and work for upto three hours at a stretch without pain. To express his gratitude, he wrote a long letter of appreciation thereafter, highlighting the efficacy of acupressure.

□

Case–34
Epileptic Fits

In the year 1999, an old patient of mine sought appointment for a patient suffering from epileptic fits. He was a 33 years old male Mr. B. When he came on the appointed date, he was accompanied by two more people to support him. Mr. B told me that he started getting the fits about seven years ago, after he had a fall from his scooter when his scooter skidded. There was no history of any head injury, bleeding from nose or ear and according to him, he had suffered only bruises in his knees and elbows. However, since then he started getting fits. He further informed that of late for the past six months or so, the incidents of fits have increased. He was not able to move alone even up to his office, which was hardly half a kilometer away from his home, and some one has to go to drop him to his office and bring him back. He was under conventional treatment and wanted to come out of it as he told that despite spending around ₹ 50,000/- to ₹ 60,000/- in tests alone, besides medicines, the problem was escalating in stead of getting any relief. He added that he feels like stopping taking the medicines being given to him by his physician. I cautioned Mr. B not to venture stopping taking medicines otherwise his condition may go out of control. Advised him to start taking acupressure treatment as a complementary therapy along with the treatment he has been taken all these years. Keep his physician informed of any changes that may come consequent upon introduction of acupressure therapy.

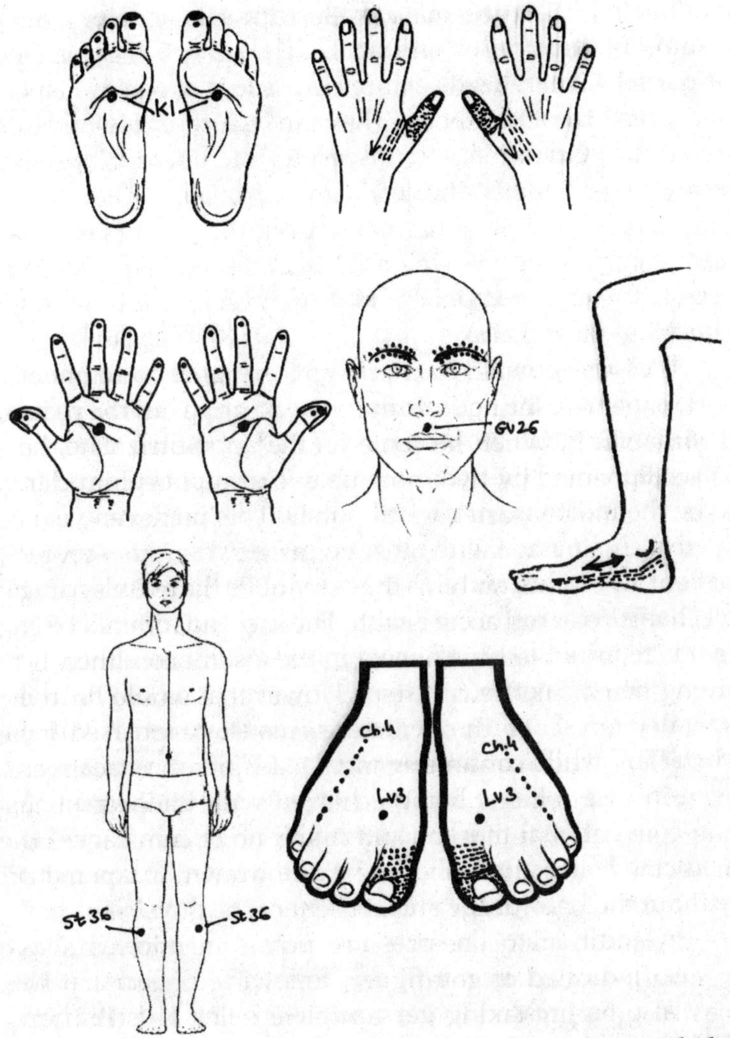

In this connection, let us first of all understand that 'epilepsy is a complex disorder of the nervous system. Irregular nerve impulses (electrical activity) in the brain can cause seizures. They may range from the person to drift off for a moment to the person falling on the floor and going into convulsions. At times the fit can be triggered by things outside the body too. It can also be defined as a sort of 'brain dysfunction'. Seizures may develop due to head injury, birth trauma, brain infection and stroke. They may be generalized or partial. Generalized seizures cause loss of consciousness and affects the whole body. They can be further divided into two forms: Grandmal seizure results into unconsciousness, entire body stiffens and jerks uncontrollably. The patient may cry, breathing becomes irregular, muscles relax and control over bowel and bladder is lost. Petitmal seizures cause momentary loss of consciousness without abnormal movements.

Pressure points in acupressure are used to re-balance and rejuvenate the body with a view to bring out the patient from fainting. Gv-26, which is located in the middle of the upper lip where the nose touches it. This point is considered to be the most potent revival points. This point can also be used in conjunction with other points, e.g. Lv-3, to revive the patient almost instantly, as they stimulate the body's natural mechanism for restoring health. The first and foremost thing that is required to be achieved in the instant condition is to strengthen the nervous system. However, it would be in the overall interest of the patient to be in constant touch with the physician, while continuing to take acupressure treatment, even in case relief is being achieved with the help of this non-conventional therapy and under no circumstances the medicine being given should be withdrawn or tapered off without the knowledge and consent of the physician.

In addition to the pressure points mentioned above as also indicated in the figure, following pressure points may also be pressed to get complete relief: K-1 (Bubbling Springs), as is evident from its name itself, which is located on the sole of the foot, between the two pads, is an important point for coming out of fainting, convulsions or shock as a result of epilepsy. Next point to be pressed is St-36, as shown in the figure, is an important point that strengthens the whole body and tones up the muscles and has been found to be of immense help in regaining consciousness.

This point when used in combination with Lv-3, which regulates and tonifies the flow of Ch'i in the liver meridian, are capable of 'Lifting the Spirits' and overcoming the emotional upsets. This combination is capable of providing relief from fainting, exhaustion caused due to the fit, nervous disorders/hangovers besides dizziness. Besides these points, pressure should also be invariably given over the reflex points pertaining to the 'Brain point' as shown in the figures, over the tip of the big toes and the thumbs of both feet and hands. Also giving pressure over the soft skin on the big toes/thumbs and the fingers which starts immediately after the nails as shown by the dotted shaded portion in those areas, with the help of some spring ring or a comb or any other object has been found to be of immense use in stimulating and strengthening the nervous and neuro system and in getting much sought after relief in the instant condition.

The patient responded very well to the therapy. Within 3-4 sessions, he reported a sense of well being. Ten sessions were given to him with out any break. Thereafter alternate days for two weeks and twice a week for next two weeks. Finally, the patient was asked to take one session every week for next two months. He was asked to keep stimulating the nervous system with the help of constant use of the spring ring almost every day for a period of three months thereafter. This patient, who was not confident to walk down alone up to his office barely 500 mtrs., after six months came to my clinic on a two wheeler scooter driving himself a distance of more than 10 kms, just to inform me that he was in good health and happy.

□

Case–35
Frozen Shoulder

In the year 2003, an old patient of mine, a very senior bureaucrat in the Govt., of India came to me with his wife who had been suffering from 'Frozen Shoulder'. This was a 54 yrs. old female Mrs. R. She told me that her problem was very old and somehow she had been managing herself at times by taking pain killers or taking resort to physiotherapy. However, she said she has got sick and tired of taking pain killers as it started showing adverse effect on her digestive system too. Besides, she said that of late her problem has become so aggravated that she finds it difficult to dress herself or comb her hair even. She confessed that earlier too her husband had told her to take acupressure treatment about two years ago, but since she was not too sure whether the therapy would be effective as she was told that during her treatment, no medicine would be given to her. She said that she could not convince herself as to how treatment could be possible without any medication. On being asked as to how she could agree for the same treatment, she confessed that she spoke to many other patients referred to me by her husband and looking into the relief they got, she also thought as to why not, as a last resort, try out this treatment also.

Here in this context, it may be mentioned that inflammation of the shoulder joint capsule is known as 'frozen shoulder'. Patient initially complains of pain in shoulder which is soon accompanied by stiffness too. Pain

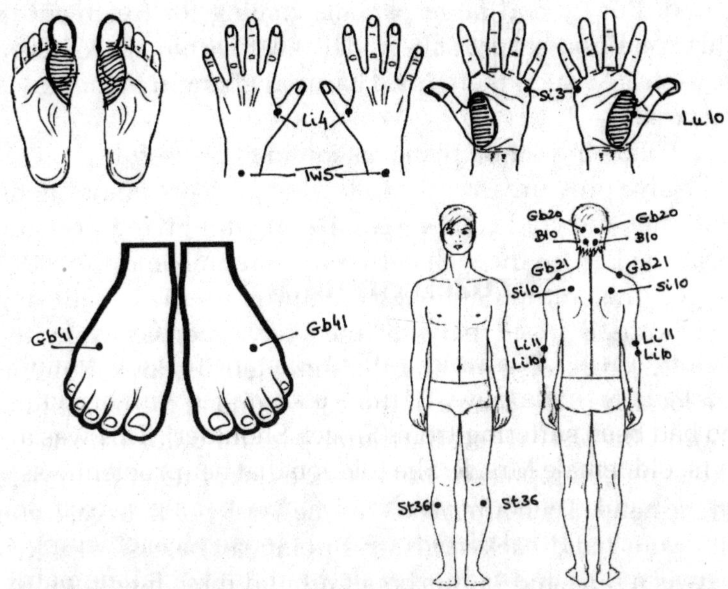

and stiffness increases for three months and thereafter remains static. The condition may worsen to the extent that the patient is not able to carry out his/her day-to-day routine, e.g. putting on/off the clothes, combing hair, normal arm movement also becomes difficult that is why the name 'frozen shoulder' has been given to this condition. The patient is not able to lift his/her arm above the elbow height, the pain radiates from neck down to the arm and across the back and chest. There may or may not be any apparent known cause. At times even minor injury to the shoulder or neglected 'cervical spondylosis' could lead to 'frozen shoulder'. Lack of movement or exercise can also be the contributory factors. It is said that this condition gets cured on its own in due course say nine months or so. But it is always better to take acupressure treatment to overcome this painful condition rather than to wait for nine months or so. For no one can say for sure that it will automatically get cured after that time period. Of course, it can't be said for sure that even with acupressure treatment it will get cured. But by and large patients coming for treatment of this condition report substantial relief within six to seven sessions. As such there is no harm in giving this therapy a fair trial.

Following action plan was found to be useful:

Give pressure over the following pressure points along with hot and cold compresses. Begin with giving pressure over the Li-4, in the web between the thumb and the index finger, this anti-inflammatory point is useful in relieving pain caused in all parts of the body, specifically in the hands, wrists, elbows, and the shoulders. Followed by Lu-10, located in the centre of the big mound at the base of the thumb, the place where the thumb joins the palm. It hurts too much on being pressed but provides lot of relief from pain in the hand. Thereafter, look for the Tw-5 point. In case you flex your hand backwards, this point can be easily located between ulna and radius bones around three finger widths from the wrist crease. Press firmly, this point removes stress from the shoulders as well as helps in getting relief from pain in the entire arm, besides toning up the muscles. Next point pressed was Li-10, just below the Li-11 point which is found over the end of the crease that is formed when you bend you hand and try to hold your shoulder. This point is also considered to be an anti-inflammatory point that helps relieve discomfort in the hands, wrists, elbow, and the shoulder joint besides giving relief to aching muscles and joints. Patients should be taught to make it a habit to stimulate this point on both the arms when they get up in the morning. Point Li-11 should be pressed very softly with modest pressure, as this point, though of great importance, gets very tender to touch, as such needs to be stimulated with great care. It relieves inflammation of the elbow and shoulder joints. Also an important point to overcome allergies of various kinds.

Followed by pressing Si-10, as shown in the figure. Press on the muscular cord of the shoulder joint. It is known to relieve arthritis, bursitis, and rheumatism. Relieves shoulder and upper back pain. Next point pressed was St-36, about four finger widths below your knee cap and one thumb width outside the shin bone. Helps in overcoming pain all over the body. It is considered to be the most potent pressure points for alleviating sore, tired muscles, and fatigue. Strengthens the whole body, tones up the muscles. Also pressed Gb-41 can be located (about two finger widths from the joint between the little and 2nd finger) above the 4th and 5th metatarsal bones. This point, besides overcoming knee pain, has been found to be of immense use in overcoming hip and shoulder tension, rheumatism, excessive water retention, and reduce stress.

After giving pressure over the reflex points discussed above, pressure was given over Gb-20, which is located in the hollow below the base of the skull to overcome stiffness in the neck and upper back pain. Followed by pressure over Gb-21, 'Shoulder Well' which lies midway between the neck and the outer edge of shoulder. This point is by and large very tender and has to be pressed very gently, simultaneously over both sides of the shoulder, the patient may be advised to take slow but deep breaths to get maximum benefit. This point restores normal flow of Ch'i in the lungs. This point should not be pressed in case of female patients, who are carrying. Next apply pressure over B-10, 'Heavenly Pillars', it is located about one and a half inches below the base of the skull, two finger widths on both side of the spine simultaneously. Relieves, headache, exhaustion, stiffness in the shoulders and swollen eyes. Si-3 is yet another point to be pressed to over come stiffness in the shoulder region, as has been shown in the figure. Press this point firmly with moderate pressure, for about a minute.

Also worked over the reflex areas of the cervical vertebrae on the big toes and the thumbs, as shown in the figure, i.e. upto the first knuckle of the thumbs and the entire big toe on both feet. Also work over the pads below the big toe and thumbs in the palms, this area reflects the scapula blades and provide lot of relief to the patients suffering from cervical problem, which may also be one of the causative factors behind frozen shoulder problem.

Since Mrs. R had told me before commencing the treatment that she would be able to take very low pressure as her pain-bearing capacity was too low. I had to give her very mild pressure for the first three to four sessions. At times with certain patients who are very sensitive to pain, we have to give absolutely mild pressure to prepare the patient mentally since once he/she starts having a feeling of well-being, they themselves ask you to increase the extent of pressure to the level of moderate pressure which is what is required. In this case too, Mrs. R told me on the 5th day that she has started having a feel that she will recover from her problem and asked me to try to increase the extent of pressure a bit but very cautiously, she said that she would herself tell me to increase in case she can bear. I raised the extent of pressure to the desired extent but she told me that she can bear a little bit more too. Actually, as the problem subsides, the extent of pain/sensitivity over the pressure point is also reduced and the patient is in a position to take more pressure. In all I gave her 15-16 sessions for about 80% recovery and thereafter asked her to discontinue the treatment to check in case her pain aggravates. But she had not to come back again. It is observed that despite stopping the sessions, the effect of acupressure treatment keeps percolating and in many cases in case you happen to meet the patient again after a month or so, they report further recovery as compared to the extent of recovery when the treatment was stopped.

□

Case–36
Obesity/Lumbago

In the year 2003, as far as I can recall, I happened to attend a case of obesity coupled with lumbago. The patient Mrs. S, was a 49-year-old female, wife of a Brigadier in Army. She was very tall, 5′7″, weight 80 kg. This case was referred to by another officer from the Army, whose wife was successfully treated some time ago.

Discussions with Mrs. S revealed that she had put on the weight in last 2-3 years since she suffered lumbago pain and had to abandon her morning and evening walks, of which she was very fond of. She also told that she had a sweet tooth. She further told me that she had also joined a much publicized weight reduction programme, spent a lot of money, but it proved to be a waste since she did loose weight there with the help of mechanical devices and dieting. But the day she stopped doing that and resorted to her normal lifestyle, she started putting on the weight and within two months after stopping going to that centre, has put on so much weight that she is 2-3 kg over and above the weight she had before joining the centre. At the outset I informed the patient that she will have to have a lot of patience in overcoming obesity, since one cannot and should not try to overcome it overnight. It is a slow process.

One point we should understand in this context is that if your body weight is 20% more than your ideal body weight or your body fat percentage exceeds 25% for male and 30% for female, you may rate yourself in the 'obese' category and

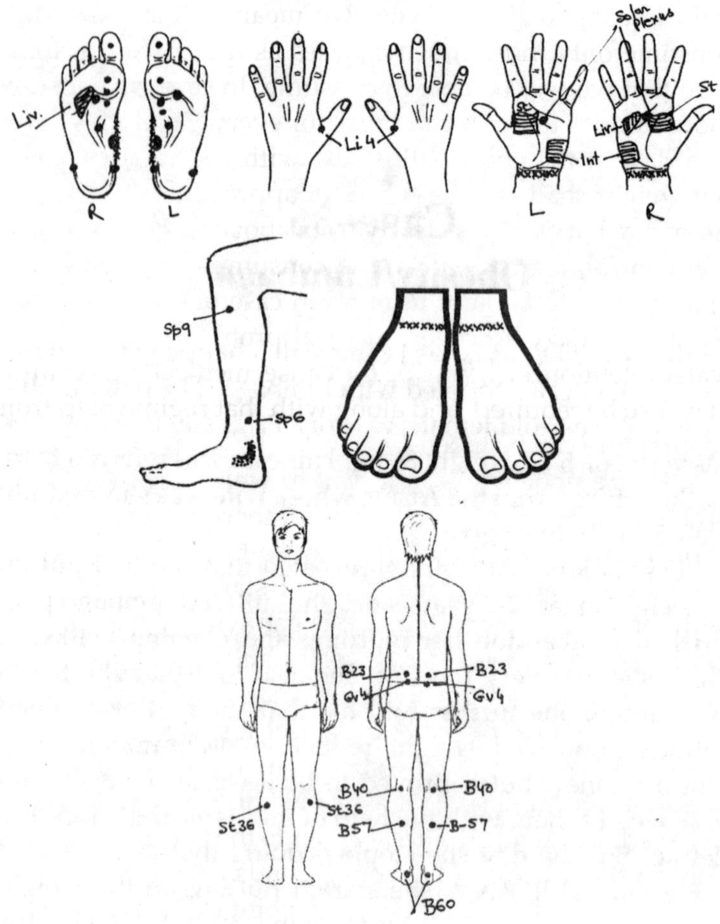

commence working upon all possible options to reduce your weight in case you do not want to run the risk of developing a heart disease, hypertension, diabetes, respiratory problem, etc. Another important thing to understand here is that although dietary restrictions shall have to be followed, yet under no circumstances, one should resort to 'fasting' alone as a means to achieve weight reduction. Another important aspect to be taken care of in handling this condition is that one should be 'calorie conscious' in case one is really serious in keeping a check over his/her weight. By coining the term 'calorie consciousness', what we mean is that we should consume only those much calories as much we can make sure that we will be able to consume. In case we consume more calories than we can burn, for every 70 calories saved in a day, at the end of 10th day, with 700 calories saved, our weight shall register a hike of approximately a pound. As such what emerges clearly from above is that exercising, diet control/regulation, calorie consumption, etc., are the main factors to be kept in mind in case one wants to beat obesity. In case, however, medical problems, e.g. thyroid, water retention, etc., may be the cause, medical intervention may also be required, and along with that regime help from acupressure can be taken.

As the patient was not able to walk due to lumbago problem, first of all, I decided to concentrate my entire effort in overcoming that problem so that Mrs. S can start her morning and evening walks. I started her treatment with the following action plan: Began with stimulating the lumbo sacral region over the soles and the palms. Direct pressure was given on the areas marked 'xxxxxx' on the lumbo-sacral part over both her feet for about 30 seconds over each reflex point as shown in figure, since giving pressure over a single reflex point for 30 seconds would have certainly made the area tender to the pressure, this was done in the fractions of 8 to 10 seconds in one go on every point thus giving pressure on one point three to four times in one session. This was followed by giving pressure over the trigger points as shown in the figure, refered to above. These are the nerve endings for the sciatic nerve in the heel of the feet, this had to be done since because of obesity there was a possibility of her sciatic nerve might have got irritated or developed some edema and could be a probable cause of excruciating pain in her back. Besides, pressure was given on the anterior and posterior sides of the heel, around the ankles on both feet, both sides as shown by the dotted lines

- the shaded portion - in clockwise as well as anti-clockwise direction and in the middle of the sole, points marked to in the figure. Patients suffering from any sort of discomfort in the lumbo sacral region respond tremendously to the points which fall on bladder meridian (B-23); B-40 (Command point) - on the back of the knee; B-57; B-60; GV-4 and Li-4, this trigger point (known as Adjoining Valley) over the large intestine meridian gives relief to pain in any part of the body by helping in circulating the Ch'i in the entire body. The precise location of these points has been shown in the figure. Within three sessions, Mrs. S reported around 15 to 20% relief. She could move within her house without much discomfort for upto 10-15 minutes.

In subsequent sessions, the following pressure points were added to the regime: These points were Sp-6, 'The Three Yin Meeting Point' which is located above the ankle bone on the inside about four finger widths, as shown in the figure. This one point stimulates the 'Yin' of three meridian, viz: kidney, liver and spleen, at the same time and is known to be perhaps one of the most important pressure point, as it helps flush Ch'i and blood through the entire body, to overcome any sort of female problem. Pressure over this point should not be given to pregnant women. Next point pressed was Sp-9, that falls on the inside of the leg, under the shin bone, just below the bulge. It reduced odema, water retention as well swelling, as also strengthens knees, an area that needed to be stimulated looking into her body weight. Further to this St-36 was pressed. This point when pressed in conjunction with Sp-6, strengthens the entire body and is also useful in quietening the rebellious Ch'i of the stomach.

In addition to above, reflex areas related to stomach, intestines, liver, pituitary, adrenals, kidneys, bladder, thyroid as well as para-thyroid, pancreas, lymphatic system as well as solar plexus are required to be stimulated by giving pressure over the reflex areas pertaining to those organs as shown in the figure at the end of this book. We also recommend

'Brisk rolling', over the foot roller which is easily available in the markets at a very nominal cost, for about three to five minutes morning and evening at least five days a week. Brisk Rolling for 3 minutes gives weightage equivalent to running two kilometers and this way weight up to two to 2-1/2 kg a month can be reduced. But please make sure that you do not resort to brisk rolling on day one itself for three minutes. Let us commence from maximum one minute for first three days and gradually increase the duration by 30 seconds every fourth day till you reach three minutes level and then go up to five minutes a day in one session.

Diet plan, as given at the end of the book, was also prescribed for Mrs. S, which she adhered to meticulously. The result was that after giving her treatment for about a month, in all around 20 odd sessions, and thereafter once a week for yet another three months, when she left Delhi along with her husband on posting, she was having four kms of morning walk, three kms of evening walk. Her weight had come down to 68 kgs. Later on her husband invited me to Agra to deliver an awareness talk on 'acupressure', to his brigade.

□

Case–37
Carpal Tunnel Syndrome (CTS)

I recall a case that came my way in the year 1998. A 34-year-old female was brought to my clinic with 'Carpal Tunnel Syndrome' (CTS) problem. She told that she has been having this problem for almost two years or so, has taken treatment at many places and every time she starts taking treatment in a different stream of science she gets some relief but that relief is too short lived and the pain and the extent of discomfort becomes intolerable again. She can't take strong pain killers as she has a new born baby to feed. She further shared that since there is no one else to support at home except her husband who has to go for work too, it becomes too difficult to manage as she finds it difficult to lift even a vessel containing one liter of milk from the gas stove as many a time it has fallen.

Carpal tunnel is a tunnel through our wrist in which tendons, arteries, veins, and nerves travel to the hands. The 'tunnel' is the cavity formed by the carpal bones and ligaments just under the skin in the wrist. This problem occurs when we make a series of similar movements, hour after hour, day after day and for months together, e.g. working on computer for long hours, playing video games, sending SMS on mobile phone very frequently, etc. The symptoms include numbness and tingling in the thumb and the first two fingers. At times the tingling spreads to the entire hand. Slowly, the thumb becomes weak and the patient is not able to hold any thing in his/her hand firmly.

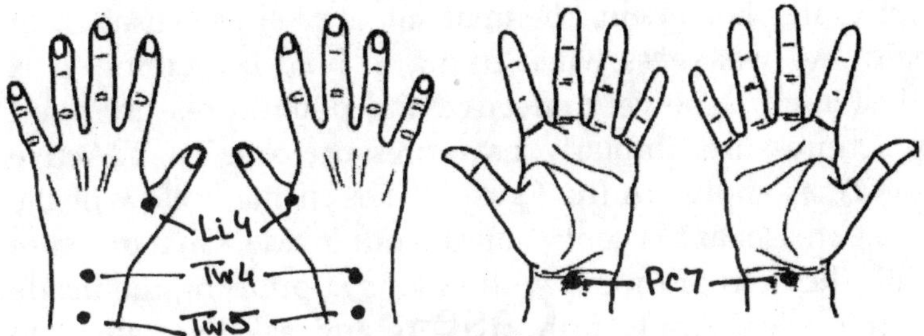

The problem may also occur due to sudden weight gain or edema, as it puts pressure over the nerves in the carpal tunnel. The problem is found in the patients suffering from arthritis too.

Pressure points technique has been found to be useful in relaxing the tendons and the muscles attached to the wrist, in alleviating pain and strengthening the thumb and the fingers in such a manner that their capability to hold things firmly is regained. The first point to be pressed was Li-4, 'Adjoining Valley'. This point is known for its ability to relieve pain, reduce inflammation and circulating the Ch'i. Pressure over this point should not be given to pregnant women. Next point pressed was Pc-6 which is known by the name 'Inner Gate'. It is located in the middle of the inner side of the forearm, 2-1/2 finger widths above the wrist crease towards the elbow. It relieves the wrist pain. Pc-7, 'the Big Mound' lies in the centre of the wrist on the palm side. Give moderate pressure over this point with the help of your thumb for about a minute to overcome the wrist pain being caused by the carpal tunnel syndrome. It helps in overcoming rheumatism and tendonitis as well to a great extent.

Next set of points to be pressed were Tw-5 and Tw-4. Whereas Tw-5 (Outer Gate) is located midway between the ulna and radius about 2-1/2 finger widths above the wrist crease, towards the elbow, on the back of the wrist. Giving pressure on this point for about a minute strengthens the wrist, alleviates pain, rheumatism as well as sensation of pain and weakness when trying to hold something. It is considered to be very effective and potent pressure point in acupressure. Similarly, gave pressure over Tw-4 (Active Pond), as shown in the figure. It lies in the hollow of the wrist crease, at the centre, on the outer side. Give pressure with the help of thumb with fingers supporting the inside of the wrist. Apply firm pressure and ask the patient to take deep and long breaths. Release gradually. Repeat the process over the other wrist too even if there is no pain there.

The patient did not respond for the first four sessions. She confessed that she was not able to give rest to her wrists at all since time and again she had to lift the child. Fortunately, next three days was a long week end and her husband was at home and he supported her. She started responding to the treatment after the sixth session, when she came for the seventh session, she was in smiles. She told me that she was able to lift vessel of milk without much discomfort. I asked her to stop coming every day and switched over to three sessions a week. In all the treatment lasted for 14 sessions.

□

Case–38
Insomnia

Around three years back in 2012, Mrs. T, aged 45 yrs., was brought to my clinic by one of my old patients, who had taken treatment from me earlier. Mrs. T had come from Paris about ten days back in connection with some business for three weeks. She told me that ever since she has come to India, she has not been able to sleep properly, partly because of Jet Leg and she said the other factor could be a bit of business stress. She was initially taken to the family physician, who had put him on to 'Alprex-0.5 mg'-HS) besides one or two more anti-depressant medicines. On proving it was revealed that the patient had a history of depression about 3-4 years back when she had suffered some losses in business. Fortunately, the patient was not too much in favour of taking medicines. (Once the patient develops the habit of taking medicines, at times it becomes extremely difficult to convince them to leave the medicines and in a way they become addicted to these medicines.)

In this connection, it may be understood that the condition in which a person gets insufficient or troubled sleep is given the name 'Insomnia' which may result into increased day time fatigue and irritability. The causative factors could be the Jet Leg (following a coast-to-coast flight); worry or mental stress; or the persons suffering from anxiety and depression may also not be able to get sound sleep. Withdrawal syndrome from hypnotic drugs may also be the cause behind insomnia. In addition going on a

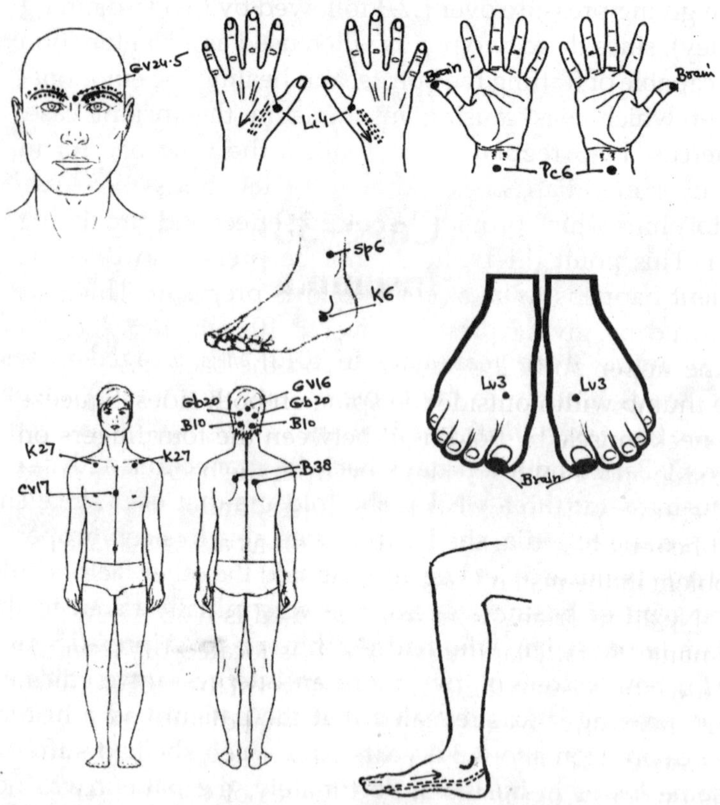

day turn from the night shift also at times becomes a reason good enough to cause this condition. Insomnia is certainly a signal given by the body of some medical condition or an emotional disturbance. A sort of fear develops in the mind of the patient as the night approaches under the apprehension that they would not be able to sleep. It becomes all the more troublesome when your partner is snoring in deep sleep and you are awake, trying hard to fall asleep.

Fortunately, acupressure has been found to be very effective in overcoming this condition. Following schedule of pressure points was followed in this case, to unblock the stagnation and rejuvenating the flow of Ch'i in the affected meridians which adversely impact the emotions. Started with giving pressure over Lv-3 followed by Li-4 (Adjoining Valley), since these two points when used as a combination are capable of 'Lifting the Spirits' and healing the emotional upset which was causing insomnia in the instant case. Whereas, Lv-3 regulates and tonifies the flow of Ch'i in the liver meridian, Li-4 is known for its ability to release endorphins which provide a soothing effect and circulating Ch'i. This point (Li-4) should not be pressed in case the patient happens to be a female and is pregnant. This was followed by giving pressure over B-10, which is located in the upper portion of the neck, on the back side, about one thumb width outside the spine on both sides. Squeeze the neck muscle by holding it between the four fingers on one side and thumb on the other, from the back. This point is the key point to over come stiffness, and combat stress and heaviness in the head, depression as also to overcome problem in the instant case.

Next important point to be pressed is B-38, known by the name, 'Vital Diaphragm' which is located between the shoulder blades and the spine at the level of the heart. It helps in relieving anxiety, grief, and emotional disturbances. Gb-20, relieves headache, stiff neck, dizziness, irritability, etc., as is evident from its name, i.e. 'Gates of Consciousness', its location is shown in the figure. It has been found to be highly beneficial in overcoming insomnia too by removing the root cause. K-27, which is located in the hollow below the collarbone next to the breast bone, also helps overcome anxiety, this point has to be pressed in case anxiety or depression is the cause behind sleeplessness. Follow this by pressing Gv-24.5, which is located between the eyebrows, as shown in figure. This tones up the endocrine system, particularly the pituitary gland, tones up the entire body, overcomes head congestion as also emotional disturbances and depression. Yet another important point to be pressed is Cv-17 (Sea of Tranquility), which is located in the centre of the breast bone. It has been found to be of immense importance in relieving nervousness, grief, depression, hysteria and other emotional disturbances. This point is highly beneficial in overcoming insomnia.

From here proceed to press Sp-6, 'The Three, Meeting Point', which strengthens the 'Yin' of kidney, liver and spleen meridians at the same time. It helps flush Ch'i and blood through the body. This combination of 'Yin' nourishing and calming effect makes is vital for getting rid of insomnia. Pc-6 which is known as 'Inner Gate' and is located on the palm side of the wrist, about three finger widths above the wrist crease in the centre of the arm, helps getting rid of insomnia by its calming effect. Next press H-7 (Spirit Gate), located on the edge of the wrist, towards the little finger side. It relieves anxiety which causes insomnia and is very helpful in this condition. Gv-16, known by the name 'Wind Mansion' is located in the centre of the head in the hollow under the base of the skull. It is known to relieve mental stress and insomnia condition. K-6 point as is evident from its very name - 'Joyful Sleep' is located below the inner side of the ankle and B-62 (Calm Sleep) as shown in the figure are also beneficial in overcoming anxiety and insomnia.

Giving pressure over the reflex area pertaining to pineal gland has also been found to be very effective in overcoming insomnia problem caused particularly because of the Jet Leg, since pineal gland controls the sleep pattern of our body. This can be followed up by giving pressure over the stress buster points over the eye brows and the brain point over the tip of the big toes and the thumbs in the feet and the hands respectively as shown in the figure as also stimulating nervous system points by giving pressure over both hands and the feet in the indicated direction.

By following the aforesaid regime of pressure points, Mrs. T, felt relieved the very first day and next day when she came for the session, reported that she fell asleep around 10.30 pm in the night but around 2.30 am she got up and thereafter she could not get sleep at all. However, she was happy that without a sleeping pill or any other medication, she could sleep for four hours . Gave her continuous sessions as she had to go back to Paris after 12 days. She came in all for 10 sessions and after the seventh session itself, she told me that she has been getting sound sleep for six to seven hours a day, which is sufficient for a healthy person. She got so much convinced about acupressure treatment that she made it a point to take at least four to five sessions every time she visited India, as a preventive. Till 2012 she visited regularly at least twice an year and whenever she had to come, she used to phone me from Paris, informing the date of her arrival and departure asking to keep time for her sessions.

In addition to giving pressure points discussed above, also recommended her to take a nice hot cup of 'tomato soup', or a glass of banana shake or hot oatmeal. What these foods have in common is that they contain a high dose of 'Melatonin', hormone that is secreted by the 'Pineal' gland in the middle of our brain. It is one of the strongest 'antioxidants' known and it is said that this hormone is full of disease curing qualities. Other foods items that are known to be rich in 'Melatonin' are sweet corn; ginger; barley; bananas and Japanese radishes. Consumption of these Melatonin rich foods an hour before bedtime would be good enough to get you a good amount of sleep without taking recourse to sleeping pills.

□

Case–39
Multiple Musculoskeletal Problems

About six months back, I happened to handle a case of a female aged about 55 years, suffering from multiple musco skeletal problems, e.g. arthritis, knee pain, stiff neck, shoulder pain, low back pain, etc. This female had been suffering for a long time and because of excessive use of pain killers, of late her digestive system had also started giving her trouble.

She had developed a sort of aversion towards food since off and on she started suffering from constipation too and straining on the toilet seat used to aggravate her body pain to intolerable levels. She was referred to me by some one around an year ago but she did not come as she had unfortunately taken 'acupressure' treatment some where and the person giving her therapy used to give her excruciating pain while giving pressure and she was terribly scared in taking acupressure treatment. Finally, she agreed to come to me when one of the common friends who had taken treatment from me told her that she will never have to complain about the extent of pain since, we never give pressure beyond the pain threshold of the patient. First day when the patient Mrs. C came, she was accompanied by her husband and one more female to support her as she was not able to walk on her own. It came to light that besides her low back pain, she had developed problem around her sciatic nerve also, as the pain was radiating from hip down to the knees too.

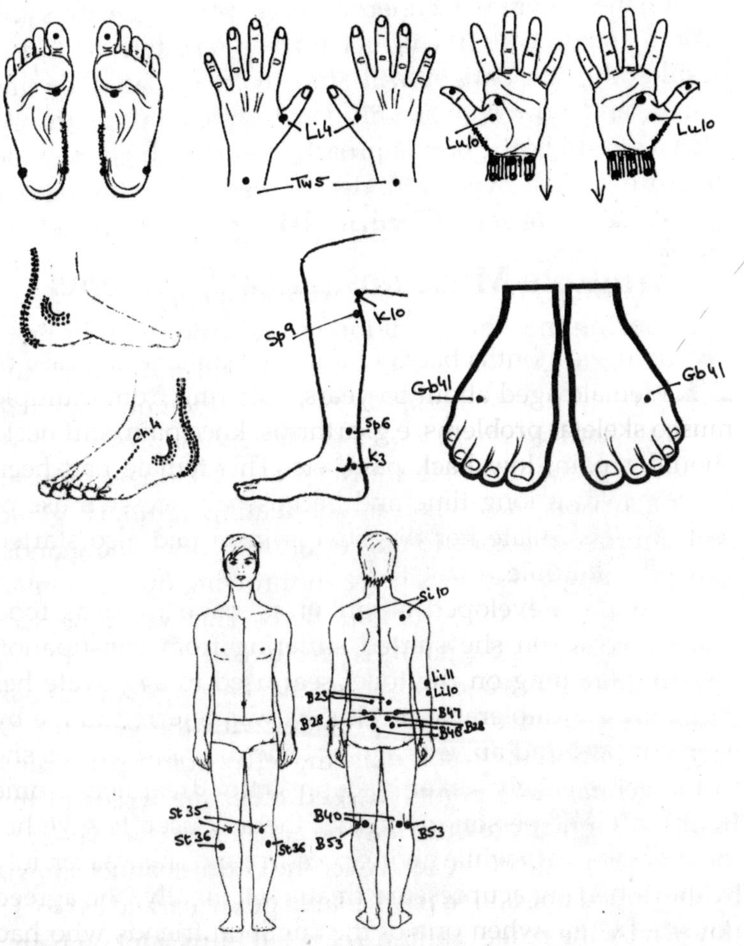

In this regard, only thing we would like to impress upon and clarify is that I have heard else where too that some therapists give very harsh pressure in their bid to give better and faster relief. This is a myth. In no way better and faster effect can be achieved by giving harsh or excessive pressure. On the contrary, on one hand it sends a wrong signal to the already suffering patient(s) and on the other hand it becomes counter productive since once a pressure point gets tender due to excessive pressure, in the next session the patient will either not allow you to give pressure over that point or it will get further sensitive to touch. Resultantly, the patient will stop treatment after getting scared, and how benefit will come without pressure. As such it would be the best approach to start with giving mild pressure, switch over to moderate pressure as the patient gets along and never be harsh in giving pressure, for getting the best results.

Following Pressure points were given to her:

Looking into the condition of the patient, I told them that for four to five sessions they should not expect any miracles and in case her body responds then only we will continue her treatment. I started with giving pressure over the point, pertaining to the 'pituitary' and, kidneys (figure), for the reason that whereas stimulating pituitary gland will improve the functioning of all the endocrine glands, strengthening of kidneys helps in throwing out unwanted accumulations (toxins) from our body. This was done over both the soles and the palms respectively.

At times it has been observed that knee and lower back pains are caused by some problem with the genitals, as such it is important to stimulate the reflex points pertaining to the genitals too, points marked other the wrists in the figure. After that pressure may be given over channel 4, i.e. the posterior side of the feet, over the entire channel shown by the dotted line and in particular at point marked as Gb-41 (known by the name 'Falling Tears'), it hurts a lot on being pressed, but this point has been found to be highly beneficial in overcoming 'knee pain', by restoring the flow of energy and thus relieves discomfort and pain in the knees.

This has to be followed by giving pressure on B-53 (Commanding Activity) and B-40 as shown in the figure Whereas B-53 is found on the outerside of the knee, B-40 lies in the middle of the back of knee, over the crease that is formed when the knee is bent. These points are highly beneficial for removing stiffness and pain in the knees.

B-54 is also usefull in alleviating 'Sciatica Pain'. Then give pressure on K-10 (Nourishing Valley), which lies on the inner edge of the knee crease, in the hollow between the two tendons and has been found to be highly effective in overcoming knee pain. Pressing Sp-9, which lies inside on the leg under the shin bone, just below the bulge, helps in reducing the edema, water retention and other discomfort in the knee area. Also press Lv-8 (Crooked Spring), which is located over the inner side of the knee, where the crease ends when knee is bent, to get relief from pain and swelling in the knees. Also press K-3; St-35 and St-36 as shown in the figure. Whereas St-35 lies in the outer indentation below the knee cap and relieves knee pain; stiffness and edema, St-36 which lies four finger widths below the knee cap, one finger width on the outside of the shin bone, is known to strengthen the whole body, tones up the muscles, particularly when used in conjunction with Sp-6, it strongly revitalizes the whole body.

After this I stimulated both soles to provide a bit of immediate relief. I gave pressure over the entire sole using 'thumb walk' technique for about 2-3 minutes, followed by giving massage like pressure over the achilles tendon area (the area behind the ankles above the heel portion), on both anterior and posterior sides of the heel. This was followed by giving pressure over the 'lumbo-sacral' area of the vertebral column, marked as 'xxxxxx' in the figure. As also point, in the same figure are the pressure points where the sciatic nerve ends over the heel. Point shown on the back of the heel is the point B-28 which pertains to the area falling over the hip joint. This point hurts a lot on being pressed but has been found to be extremely beneficial in overcoming any sort of discomfort in the lower back area.

Then gave pressure on B-23 point, as shown in the figure. This point has been found to be of immense help in alleviating lower back pain, sciatica, and fatigue caused due to severe pain in that area. This was followed by giving pressure over B-47, as shown, this point when pressed in conjunction with B-23, helps a lot in providing relief in the pain in the low back region besides helping in overcoming fatigue, fear as also calming down the irritated sciatic nerve. Further to this, I pressed B-48, which helps provide relief in sciatica, hip pain, lower back pain and in alleviating tension in the region. This was followed by giving pressure over the following pressure points. Began with giving pressure over the Li-4, in the web between the thumb and the index finger, this anti-inflammatory point is useful in relieving pain caused by arthritis in all parts of the body, specifically in the hands, wrists, elbows, and the shoulders. Followed by Lu-10, located in the centre of the big mound at the base of the thumb, the place where the thumb joins the palm. It hurts too much on being pressed but provides lot of relief from pain in the entire arm. Thereafter look for the Tw-5 point. In case you flex your hand backwards, this point can be easily located between ulna and radius bones around three finger widths from the wrist crease. Press firmly. This points removes stress from the shoulders as well as helps in getting relief from pain in the entire arm, besides toning up the muscles. Next point pressed was Li-10, just below the Li-11 point which is found over the end of the crease that is formed when you bend you hand and try to hold your shoulder (figure). This point is also considered to be an anti-inflammatory point that helps relieve arthritic discomfort in the hands, wrists and the elbow joints besides giving relief to aching muscles and joints due to arthritis. Arthritic patients should be taught to make it a habit to stimulate this point on both the arms when they get up in the morning. Point Li-11 should be pressed very softly with modest pressure, as this point, though of great importance, gets very tender to touch, as such needs to be stimulated with great care. It relieves inflammation of the elbow and shoulder joints. Also an important point to overcome allergies of various kinds.

To end the session, pressed Si-10, as shown in the figure. It lies on the muscular cord of the shoulder joint. It is known to relieve arthritis, bursitis, and rheumatism. Relieves shoulder and upper back pain. After having given pressure as stated above pressed B-47, which is located on the lower back between second and third lumber vertebrae about 1-1/2" away from spine on its both sides. It relieves lower backaches and fatigue.

At the end of the session, when I asked her to get up, she said she will have to wait till her husband comes as she would not be able to get up on her own. When her husband came, she was pulled from both hands by her husband and her attendant. But this had to done only for five sessions. As matter of fact after the fourth session itself, she could lift her leg without support. Otherwise, she used to lift her leg with the help of both of her hands for putting her leg over the stool to take pressure. When she came for the seventh session, she complained of escalation of pain in the back and shoulders. But her husband, who used to accompany her told her to tell the entire thing and not only about the increase in pain. Then she shared that after taking the sixth session, when she went down, she felt that she can walk. She asked her husband to take her to the mall, where she went around for about an hour. Probably, the exertion resulted into aggravation. I advised her to start moving within her house for the present and only gradually increase the duration and distance. It took her about 24 sessions for recovery to the extent that she started working in her kitchen as well and attending her day-to-day activities as before without much discomfort. She was also advised to adhere to some diet plan, that has been given in the end of this book for patients suffering from musco-skeletal disorders.

□

Case–40
Irritable Bowel Syndrome (IBS)

During the year 2002, an old patient of mine who belonged to the Indian Police Service, introduced me to his junior colleague who has been suffering from certain problems of the digestive system. He was around 46 yrs. of age. His symptoms included alternating diarrhea and constipation, excessive flatulence, loss of appetite and an overall feeling of weakness. He informed that at times he gets cramps also in his abdomen. He had been suffering from this problem for the past three to four years, when he was posted in North East region. Had tried treatment in almost every stream of science, but was not getting total relief. In between, he informed, he used to get some relief, but soon the symptoms would reappear. All this was despite the fact that he had been exercising almost regularly and had been trying to avoid going to parties also to the extent possible. He was a non-smoker and non-alcoholic. This disease is known by the name "Irritable Bowel Syndrom" (IBS).

Although there is no known cause of this condition, it is believed that stress and autonomic nervous system which responds to stress may be the cause behind. Certain foods too irritate the bowel. According to TCM, imbalance in 'Earth Energy' in our body may cause this disease. According to them, in case out of the five vital elements of our body, if your system is dominated by the earth element, you may have the tendency to overeat and this may also cause problem. Some people suffering from this condition

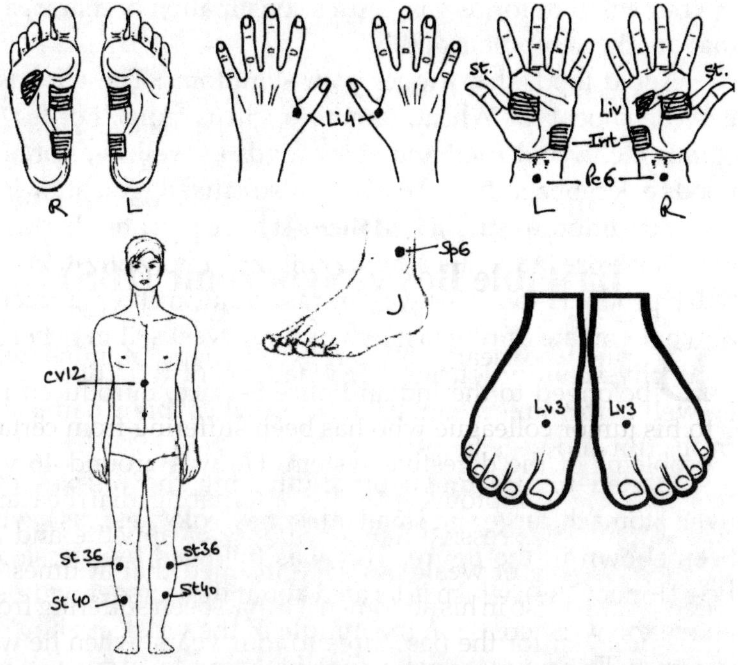

also tend to put on weight. They develop craving for sweets, chocolates, etc., which further add to the problem. Other conditions that cause burning in the stomach and chest, bloating, distension after eating, belching and difficulty in swallowing food, etc., include non-ulcerative dyspepsia, gastritis, and peptic ulcers, etc. An additional cause of this sort of digestive problem may be the invasion of microscopic pests (bacteria). The ideal solution would be to get your dietary routine regulated in consultation with some dietician.

Drinking enough water at least 8 to 12 glasses, avoid fatty foods, eat well-cooked food as raw food puts more strain on your spleen, an organ responsible for breaking down and extracting essential nutrients from food. Soups and stews are considered to be good spleen nourishing foods. Experts recommend maintaining a food diary so that you are able to keep a track as to which food triggers a painful spasm in your colon or forms gas, causes constipation or diarrhea, that are the symptoms of IBS.

Avoid foods that trigger your symptoms. These foods may be chocolate. Wheat, tomatoes, citrus fruits, hot tea/ coffee, etc. Avoid fried and spicy foods as well as alcohol. Foods e.g. cabbage, nuts, beans can also cause aggravation in your condition, as such avoid them. In case you are a known case of lactose intolerance, avoid/minimize consumption of dairy products too. This way in case you can keep a track of what you ate during last two or three weeks, it may help your physician in figuring out what sort of food does not go well with your system. Eat more of wheat bran, oatmeal, fresh fruit and vegetables.

Started his treatment by stimulating the reflexes of liver, stomach, large and small intestines, colon, etc., as have been shown in the figure. This was followed by pressing Pc-6 (Inner Gate), which is located about three finger widths above the wrist crease in the middle of the wrist, as shown in figure. This point is known to relieve nausea, in particular which troubles the patient of IBS, due to its calming effect. Next point to be pressed was Li-4, 'Adjoining Valley', the point which lies in the web between the thumb and the index finger. It improves the intestinal activity besides relieving abdominal distention and also constipation that leads to the formation of gas.

Next, I gave pressure over St-36 (Three Mile Point) as shown in the figure. This point also relieves indigestion, prevents gas formation and bloating. Moderate yet firm pressure needs to be given over this point. You will find that most of the time I have followed point Sp-6, 'Three Meeting Point' immediately after pressing St-36. The reason behind is that by doing so the effectiveness of both these points multiplies manifolds. As such make it a point that pressure over this combination has to be given in conjunction to drive maximum benefit out of them.

However, make sure that pressure over Sp-6 is not gı to pregnant women.

Further, gave pressure over Lv-3, as shown in figure to overcome stress and thereby get relief from distention, nausea, vomiting, and abdominal pain too that is, at times, caused due to distention. Followed by giving pressure over Cv-12, as shown to overcome indigestion, heartburn, abdominal pain, constipation besides helping in restoring the balance in earth energy to overcome IBS. As also St-40, which is located half way between the ankle bone outside of the foot and centre of the knee cap, as shown. It is very useful for reducing congestion as also in overcoming the imbalance in 'Earth Energy' which is the prime cause of Irritable Bowel Syndrome according to TCM.

When the patient Mr. S, came for the fifth session, he told me that perhaps his body is responding well to this treatment. He added that for past two days the extent of discomfort has registered noticeable change. I told him to switch over to sessions on the alternate days with a view to increase the span of treatment without increasing the number of sessions. In all 14 sessions did the job. Mr. S was too happy. Thereafter, I kept in touch with him for more than four years. He even engaged me to attend patients in the MI room in his para-military force in which he enjoyed a commanding position. During this period, he never had to come back for his IBS problem at all.

□

Case–41
Binge Eating Disorders (BED)

I recall of a case of Mrs. C, age 52 years, height 5′3″, with symptoms of eating disorder. She complained that about four years ago, after she attained menopause, she developed a tendency to put on weight. Her weight increased from 58 kgs to 67 kgs. As her husband who was an Army Officer was very particular about his own weight as well as that of his wife, on the recommendation of some common friend, she resorted to 'dieting'. She further reported that her dietician put her under rigorous dieting plan and she was kept fasting; over soups and boiled vegetables for quite some time.

Though she succeeded in shedding her weight to a great extent, (her weight came down to 61 kgs within a period of a month), yet after that when she tried to come back to her normal routine, she found that she has developed a very peculiar symptom. At times she felt that she has developed a disliking for normal food, a case of loss of appetite. Even the smell of food made her feel nauseatic, whereas at times she felt that she has started involving herself in binge eating. She further added that, at times, while swallowing she feels discomfort as if she has to put extra effort in swallowing the food but now for about a week or so, the problem has got aggravated to the extent that she has to drink a draught of water to swallow the food.

Eating disorders, whether mild or binge eating disorders (BED) should not be ignored as they could take

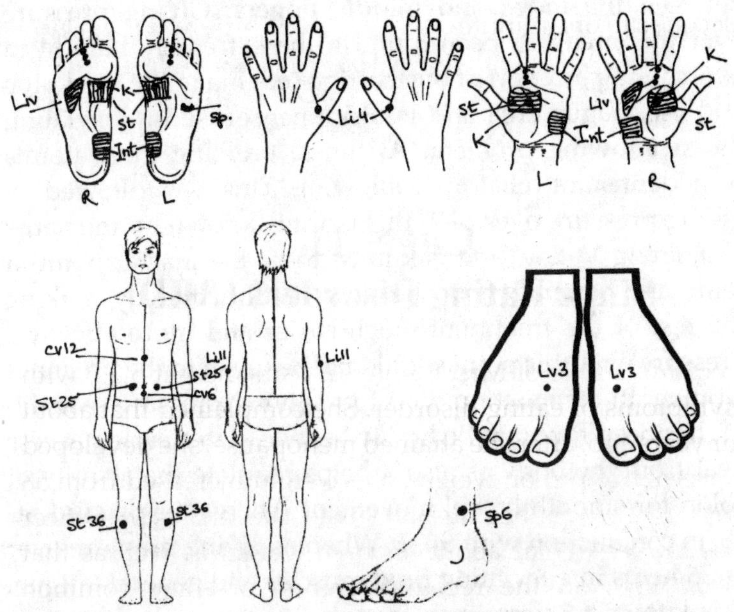

a serious turn in case not attended to timely. Though this could be age related also, but this could happen at any age which at times leads to loss of appetite. Researches have found that 'eating disorder' may also be caused by 'strict dieting' control as this could cause the brain chemicals to go haywire. According to them, the deprived feeling in respect of certain foods might also trigger BED. As such the moment you suspect that you are suffering from eating disorder, you should immediately get in touch with your physician/dietician as the management may require a healthy diet besides counseling.

The following regime of acupressure points was adopted:

To begin with stimulated the zones of pressure points relating to the liver, stomach, large and small intestines, etc., so as to improve the functioning of each of them, as shown in the figure in both the soles and the palms. There after pressure was given in the area depicted by three '***', between the index and middle fingers. Giving pressure over this area has been found to be extremely helpful in overcoming any sort of obstruction/edema in the food pipe and esophagus area and is of immense use in alleviating the swallowing problem. At times, pressing these points provide instant relief in swallowing. This was followed by giving pressure over Li-4, this point is known by the name 'Adjoining Valley' and is known to be the master point in removing stagnation in the flow of Ch'i thereby making the rest of the treatment much easier and more effective. Pressure over this point should not be given to the pregnant women. In conjunction with Li-4, giving pressure over Li-11, has been found to be highly beneficial in clearing excess heat from the body as also it helps regulate the activity of colon for smooth bowel movement. Thereafter pressed St-36, in conjunction with Sp.-6. Whereas giving pressure over St-36 helps in alleviating tired muscles and general fatigue, it is known to strengthen the whole body, aids digestion, and relieves stomach disorders by stimulating intestinal functioning. Giving pressure over Sp-6, the 'Three Yin Meeting Point' located above the ankle bone towards the inside of the leg on the back side, is known to be one of the best points since it strengthens three meridians, viz. kidneys, liver and spleen at the same time and helps flush the Ch'i and blood through the body. Thereafter, I gave pressure over Cv-6 and Cv-12 points. Whereas Cv-6, known as 'Sea of Energy' is located three finger widths below the naval and is known to relieve abdominal pain, colitis and gas formation, Cv-12, as its name 'Middle Stomach' itself suggests is located midway between the breast bone and the belly button. The famous combination of Cv-6; Cv-12 and St-25 which is known as 'Four Doors' is highly beneficial to overcome any type of stomach or gastrointestinal disorders, including 'BED'. This was followed by giving pressure over St-25, which is located two thumb widths from the vertebral column on both sides, at the back of belly button. Pressure over this point has to be given on both sides simultaneously with medium yet firm pressure for 30 seconds to one minute to get best results. To end the session, pressed Lv-3, as shown in the figure, this point is known to regulate and tonify the liver and the flow of Ch'i in the liver meridian and is known to provide relief in almost all the symptoms connected with the digestive system.

Besides the above treatment, she was asked to read the book, *Food and Mood* written by Elizabeth Somer, M.A., R.D. in which she has outlined the need to focus on a healthy and balanced eating lifestyle, excerpts of which are reproduced below:

Reduce the fat in your diet to 25% of calories.

Limit sugars to 10% or less of your total calories.

Limit caffeine to two servings or less.

Eat at least three servings of fruit; four servings of vegetables; seven servings of breads and grains, and one serving of legumes.

Divide calories evenly between five or six small meals a day. Eat a meal or snack every four hours.

Take a vitamin/mineral supplement if you are not eating at least 2500 calories a day from a variety of nutritious foods.

In addition, she has recommended that you always eat breakfast, and drink at least eight glasses of water every day. She further recommends that changing your habits slowly, and not in one shot, will give your body and brain chemicals time to adjust.

Further, in a study, researchers have found that those who switched to nutritious and low sugar diets got relief from binges within three weeks. As such, based on what has been stated above, try and follow the below mentioned tips:

Instead of dieting, take recommended amount of calories.

Cut on caffeine, to minimize your risk of binge eating.

Take many small meals rather than eating two or three times a day.

Follow a time schedule for eating, as far as possible.

Include fruits, vegetables and whole grain breads in your diet plan.

Make sure that you consume adequate vitamins and minerals and maintain proper zinc levels in your body, as the deficiency may lead to interference with your taste and smell buds.

Mrs. C responded well to the treatment and also supported in changing her food habits as well as intake gradually. In all 14-15 sessions were given to her to get the desired results.

□

Case–42
Disc Prolapse

I recall of handling the case of a lady doctor (physician) who was herself running a private clinic, her husband was also a senior physician in one of the well-known hospitals. The patient was bed ridden for about a week as she had suffered a prolapsed disc. The problem further aggravated as she had to lie down in her bed all the time in a particular position and as such developed 'wry neck' too. She was really in tremendous pain and the treatment she was getting was total bed rest as also pain killing shots. Somehow, a colleague of her father who happened to know me told him to contact me for his daughter's treatment. But, unfortunately, neither the patient nor her husband who were young medicos had no faith in any thing else except the stream of science they had studied were perhaps not too sure about perusing the treatment under going acupressure therapy. But, somehow, the father of the patient persuaded them to try when she was not getting any relief, they agreed. When they approached me, I told them that I can go to their residence, but since I did not want to waste my time in locating their house, I requested them to arrange for my pick up and dropping. Dr. A, the patient's husband came on his own to pick me. While going to their place, obviously he was very inquisitive, wanted to know lots about what I was going to do, etc. I too took the complete history of the case from him so as to save time of both of us. He informed me that the extent of pain was so much that she was not able

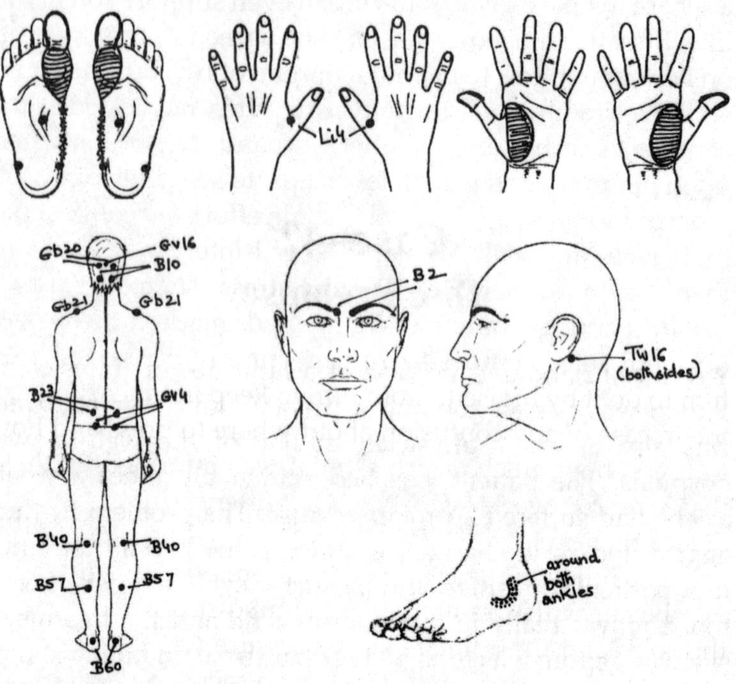

even to turn in the bed, was being given bed pan for passing urine and stool.

On reaching home, I straightaway started giving pressure to her. After attending her for around 30-35 minutes, I requested her to try to sit on her bed. The patient almost screamed at me saying has my husband not told you what sort of problem I have been facing? She added that you have not given any injection or pain killer, how you can imagine that I will be able to sit? I could understand and appreciate her anxiety since she had no faith or exposure to this sort a treatment earlier. I told her that I have attended her for more than half an hour and did she think I had to settle any thing with her that I had been giving her more pain by pressing various pressure points. Somehow, her husband who had been told about acupressure while on our way to their home, told her to try when I was so confident. He said both of us are here to take care of you, we can even support you if you like. But after much persuasion, she agreed to try to get up on her own. It took her about a minute of two but she could sit herself with some maneuvering. This inculcated some confidence in her and also her husband. Now he insisted upon her to try and walk a few steps, to see if she can walk too. And to their surprise, after some effort she could stand by herself and walk 4-5 steps. Now I intervened and told them not to put her body to more stress. Thereafter, I told her husband the points to be pressed, marked them over her both soles, left an instrument (jimmy) there and told him to do it by himself. I told him to keep in touch, and ask me in case of any confusion about where to press and how to press, how much to press, etc. I was informed by them that within a week's time she was fit enough and started attending her clinic.

The following pressure points were pressed:

Began with stimulating the lumbo sacral region over the soles and the palms. Direct pressure was given on the areas marked 'xxxxxx' on the lumbo-sacral part for about 30 seconds over each reflex point as shown in figure, since giving pressure over a single reflex point for 30 seconds would have certainly made the area tender to the pressure, this was done in the fractions of 8 to 10 seconds in one go on every point thus giving pressure on one point three to four times in one session. This was followed by giving pressure over the other trigger points marked in the figure, refered to above. These are the nerve endings for the sciatic nerve in the heel of the feet. Besides, pressure was given on the anterior and posterior sides of the heel, around the ankles on both feet, both sides as shown by the dotted lines - the shaded portion - in clockwise as well as anti-clockwise direction and in the middle of the sole, points marked in the figure. Patients suffering from any sort of discomfort in the lumbo sacral region respond tremendously to the points which fall on bladder meridian (B-23); B-40 (Command

Point), on the back of the knee; B-57; B-60; Gv-4 and Li-4, this trigger point (known as Adjoining Valley) over the large intestine meridian gives relief to pain in any part of the body by helping in circulating Ch'i in the entire body. The precise location of these points has been shown in the figure.

As for providing relief for the 'wry neck', I pressed at Gv-16 (Wind Mansion) which is located in the hollow under the base of the head. This relieves stress and stiffness in the neck. Followed by B-2 (Drilling Bamboo) which lies in the indentation over the bridge of the nose between the eyebrows to get relief in neck pain, fatigue, and headache if any. Next I pressed Gb-20 (Wind Pool) which is located on both sides of the spine of your neck, about a thumb width over the hairline, in the depression, at the base of the skull. Gb-21 (Shoulder Well) is located midway between the neck and outer edge of the shoulder. It restores the normal flow of Ch'i and is very helpful in reducing shoulder tension and fatigue. Thereafter pressed B-10 (Heavenly Pillars), this point can be pressed by holding the neck from behind clinching between four fingers joined on one side and the thumb on the other. It helps overcome stress and stiff neck (wry neck). To end the session, I gave pressure over Tw-16 which lies in the indentation at the base of the skull, approx., two inches on the back of the earlobe, as shown in the figure, to get relief in stiff neck and reduce pain in shoulder and neck.

□

Case–43
Pre-Menstrual Syndrome (PMS)

This case is being quoted, not as any specific case history, but in view of the fact that at least 25 to 50% women who have not yet reached the menopause stage suffer from Pre-Menstrual Syndrome (PMS). We have been successful in mitigating the sufferings of hundreds of females who confront this condition, some time or the other during their life time, by adopting certain lifestyle interventions in the form of exercising, food habits and of course using acupressure technique. Following the given tips shall prove to be a boon to the women, suffering from PMS.

We all know that menstrual cycle is a natural process in women, which is associated with pain or discomfort, both physiological and psychological. The extent of discomfort or pain, of course, varies in each individual. The symptoms present in the shape of tenderness in the breast(s); water retention; irritability; weight gain or mood swings, etc. Whereas most of the women accept this melody as a part of their life, yet it has been noticed that those with sedentary lifestyle, who do not take regular walks, exercise or eat a balanced diet suffer more than those who follow a proper lifestyle.

As a matter of fact, it is the imbalance in the Ch'i of the Liver meridian and its stagnation that is the prime cause behind this condition. The entire liver meridian including the main organ is responsible for initiating the menstrual cycle. Following the schedule of pressing the

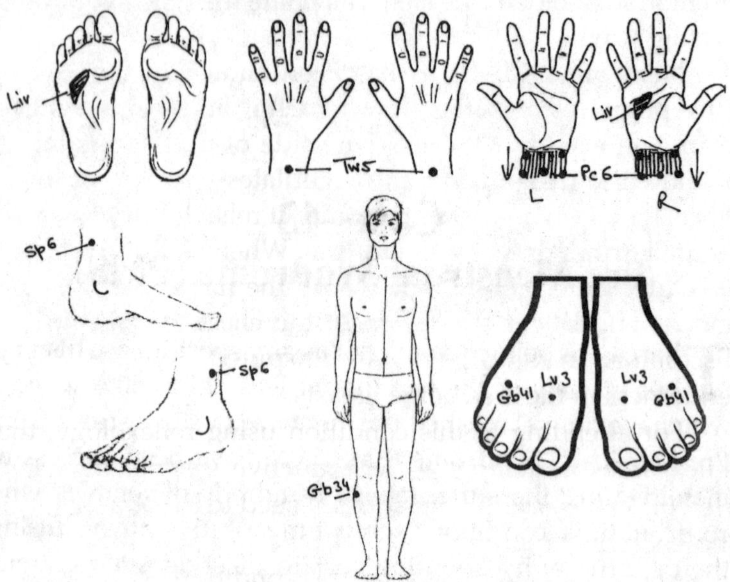

follows pressure points has been found to be very helpful in overcoming the pain and discomfort caused. Adopt this schedule as a part of your self help programme, at least four times during the first two three weeks and there after at least 7 to 10 days before the MC date every alternate day. These points should not be pressed during the cycle or once a lady has conceived.

Lv-3, as shown in the figure, is known to regulate and tonify the Liver and the flow of 'Ch'i in the liver meridian and is known to provide relief in almost all symptoms to the patient undergoing the transition period of menopause.

Gb-20, known by the name, 'Gates of Consciousness', located below the base of skull, in the hollow space, as shown in figure. It is extremely helpful in overcoming stress, mood swings, and irritability.

Sp-6, 'Three Ying Meeting Point', is a crucial point to be pressed for almost any female problem(s) as it strengthens the 'Yin' of three meridians, viz. kidneys; liver and spleen at the same time. Helps stimulate Ch'i in the entire body and circulation of blood too. Helps alleviate the PMS symptoms in a big way.

Next press Gb-41, as has been shown in the figure. This point restores the flow of Ch'i, and helps relieve PMS. Followed by Gb-34 (Sunny side of the Mountain). It is known to dispel wind and stimulates the 'Yin' of liver. Since liver's yin nourishes the joints, it relieves the muscular strain. Further press Tw-5 and Pc-6. Whereas, Tw-5 (known as 'Outer Gate'), Pc-6 is known by the name 'Inner Gate', and its effect over the region of the chest for any sort of discomfort, in that region, is undisputed. Overcomes the tenderness in the area of the breasts.

For attending to this condition using reflexology, the reflex areas pertaining to reproductive system, digestive system, kidneys, endocrine glands need to be stimulated as shown in the figure.

Many patients affected by this condition report certain cravings in their food habits in particular. The cravings could be of the sort of desire for chocolates, cookies, or for aerated drinks (sugars). However, it has been noticed that fulfilling these cravings may prove to be more problematic later on as it could result into weight gain, water retention or mood swings, the other associated symptoms of PMS. As such avoid satisfying such cravings and concentrate on: protein/fiber rich food, carbohydrates like potatoes, whole grain breads, these will relieve your cravings and provide a better frame of mind. Fish high in Omega-3 might reduce PMS symptoms.

Another good source of Omega-3 could be 'Oat germ', salmon, tuna or white fish. Spinach, broccoli, sweet potatoes are rich in 'beta carotene' which is converted into Vitamin A, that helps alleviate the discomfort PMS causes. Consumption of Vitamin B6 could help overcome fatigue, depression, breast pain, water retention mood swings, and sleep pattern. Good source of Vit. B6 could be: Green leafy vegetables, chicken, beans, etc. Similarly, calcium consumption will be found to be helpful in reducing depression, back pain, irritability and headaches associated with this condition.

Further, add a little bit of magnesium (around 300 mg a day) to your diet, to overcome nausea, cravings, mood swings, cramps, and headache. The source could be nuts, peas, spinach, broccoli, and seafood. Also based on some studies conducted it has been found that even a minor drop in level of 'zinc' might trigger the PMS. As such do not forget to add foods like black beans, lima beans, oysters or turkey, etc., to replenish the deficiency of zinc if any.

Among the ancient herbs, the herbs that can bring magnificent relief in PMS symptoms are chaste tree, which is known for ages to overcome any sort of female problems. The extract brings back the progesterone and estrogen levels into balance, thereby relieving the PMS symptoms. Ginkgo is another herb known for centuries and is known to alleviate PMS symptoms particularly the breast pain. Parsley is yet another herb which is loaded with Vit. C and researches have shown that it has great potential for overcoming pre-menstrual pains.

Yoga tips given at the end of the book can also prove to be a boon for the female who have suffered a lot from this condition. Adopt them and see for yourself the difference it makes.

□

Case–44
Osteoporosis

About two years ago, a friend of mine, who has also been practising the art and science of acupressure, phoned me to discuss the case of one Mrs. B, aged about 59 years. He shared with me that the lady was bed-ridden since she had been suffering from "osteoporosis" for almost 20 years. The female also had many other problems like incontinence, asthma, and hiccups besides very low immunity as she was having a poor digestion too. On the whole, it looked like a challenging case, since the patient had lost interest in life as she had suffered a lot. He as hardly willing to take any treatment and when I spoke to her over phone, she told me, "Doctor, I am sure my problems have no end. Can you help me in getting me rid of this life? "………. After much persuasion from his family members, who had some good experience with acupressure treatment in their own family under our care, she agreed to be under our care.

Here, it may be desirable to mention that the word, 'osteoporosis' means 'porous bones'. In this condition, the bones gradually weaken and get prone to getting fractured. In advanced cases, even a tough sneeze or vigorous coughing may cause a fracture in the ribs or any other part of the body. It has been observed that the most-affected part(s) of the body that are affected are ribs, hip joint, spine or even the wrist. Neck of the femur is the worst affected area. Further, this condition is prevalent more in female than in male, more so after the woman undergoes the process of menopause, as

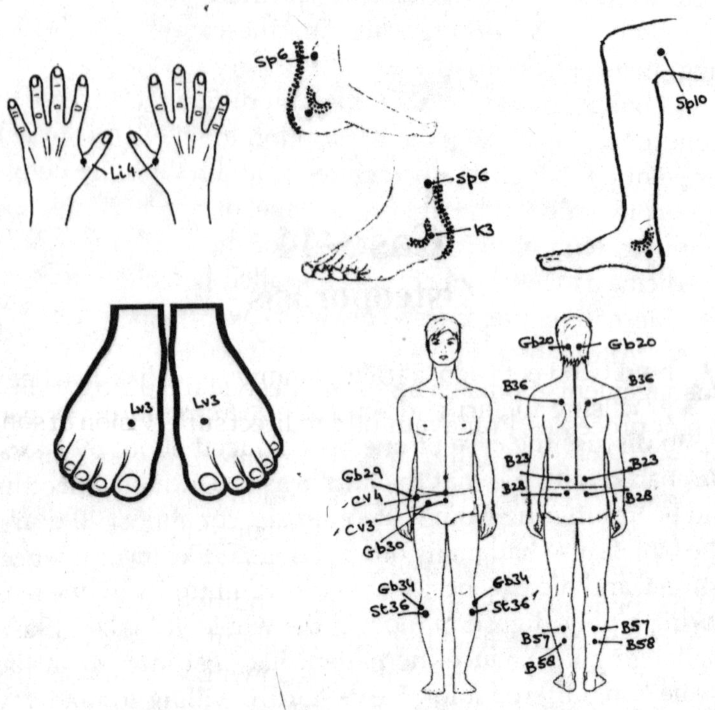

the body undergoes hormonal changes, thereby resulting into loss of bone density. In males, the incidence/intensity of this disease is comparatively much lesser.

The exact causative factor responsible for this condition is not known. However, it has been seen that around 35-40 years of age, the bones begin to lose calcium, the vital most element required for the bones. After menopause, the production of estrogen that maintains the calcium content in the bones is substantially reduced. No doubt that loss in bone density is attributable partly to ageing factor too, but hereditary factor cannot be ruled out all together. The incidence of this ailment is found more in the women whose ovaries had to be removed by or before attaining the age of 40 years or so. It is said that the risk factor for suffering from this condition, in such women, is as high as four times when compared with others. As hyperthyroidism and kidney problems adversely affect the capacity of the body in absorbing calcium, these ailments further aggravate osteoporosis.

Looking at the fact that it is a bit difficult to reverse the condition, it is always the best option to take a recourse to prevention, which is much easier to attain with the help of non-conventional therapies that have, of late, become more popular, with growing awareness of the side effect of the medicine as well as upcoming so-called holistic treatments or alternative therapies. However, we try to shun this term 'Alternative Therapy' and advocate the term 'Co-management'. Some changes in Lifestyle (resorting to light Yogic processes, Pranayam under direct supervision of some Yoga expert), following strict diet control, i.e. consumption of some vegetables/fruits (information provided at the end of the book), as well as following acupressure/reflexology have shown much improvement in mitigating the sufferings of the patients suffering from this condition.

After counseling the patient about certain life style changes in her eating habits, following the schedule of pressure points as discussed below was found to be of immense use in the case under discussion:

At the outset, it may be mentioned, as a caution, that extremely mild pressure has to be given to the patients suffering from osteoporosis. May be till the therapist is not sure about the intensity of the bone density loss, merely massage-like pressure over the prescribed pressure points is recommended, since a mild excess pressure in those areas may do more damage than any benefit to the patient. As such, we repeat that extremely mild pressure should be given to such patients.

To begin with, press "St-36 that lies four-finger width below the knee cap, one-finger width on the outside of the shin bone. This point strengthens the whole body, tones up the muscles. Particularly when pressed in combination with Sp-6, it strongly revitalises the whole body and has been found to be specifically beneficial in female patients. All that is required is to press both of these points one after the other in continuation, irrespective of the fact that which point of the two is pressed first. As the name given to Sp-6 suggests that it is called 'Three Yin Meeting Point', it is located about four-finger widths above the ankle bone on the inner side. It strengthens three vital organs of our body, e.g. kidney, liver, and spleen. It helps flush Ch'i and blood through the body. Pregnant women should not press this point.

Next point pressed was GV 24.5. This point is located over the bridge of the nose, where eyebrows and the bridge of the nose meet and is appropriately known by the name. 'The Third Eye'. This point stimulates and balances the pituitary gland, the master endocrine gland and, thus, helps in stimulating and correcting the functioning of thyroid and para-thyroid glands too, thereby helping in maintaining the calcium requirement in our body. The next point pressed was Lv-3. It regulates and tonifies the functioning of the liver and consequently the flow of Ch'i in the liver meridian. This point is also known for its ability to grossly improve the immunity in human body, besides being helpful in detoxification as well as improving the health of gallbladder.

Further to this, press the point 'Adjoining Valley', Li-4 which is known for its efficacy in mitigating pain and improving circulation of Ch'i, as also overcome stagnation. This point too is known for its ability to eliminate toxins out of our body through bowels. Pregnant women should not take pressure over this point. Futher, press K-3, a point that lies between the inside of the ankle bone and the achilles tendon in the back of the ankle. It helps overcome stress over the genitals, stimulates kidneys and regulates menstrual irregularities. Next to this, press Th-13, a point that lies on the back of upper arm, below the shoulder. This point is capable of taking care of the functioning of the thyroid gland, infections of the lymph passages in the neck, throat and armpit. It has been found to be very effective in prevention of osteoporosis. Similarly, Si-10, which is just below Si-9, i.e. below the upper edge of the shoulder blade, helps in lymph drainage problems in the throat and neck area. Next press Li-14, which is approximately seven-thumbs width above the Li-11, on the outside of the upper arm. This point has also been found to be of much help in the condition under discussion.

For the prevention and cure of this condition using reflexology, stress was laid on the reflex areas pertaining to pituitary, uterus, ovaries, chest, and lungs. Please note that pressure is given to such patients only with the help of thumbs and fingers and no probe like Jimmy should be used so that very mild and balanced pressure is given. Please refer to the pictures of palms and soles at the end of the book to refer to the reflex areas pertaining to various organs as listed above.

Further to above, handling the patient suffering from this condition, using Naturopathy, Ayurvedic way, the practitioner would recommend you dietary modifications, herbal medicines and exercises that include breathing techniques, yoga postures, daily walks, etc. Food is very much a medicine for osteoporotic bones. Soy products, soaked almonds, white sesame seeds, yogurt and aloe in specific quantities at specific time may be required. As such, food combinations are to be carefully selected not only for the nutrients but also to enhance the uptake of minerals and vitamins for the body.

Magnets are really remarkable for mitigating pains.... This is achieved by placing magnets over the area of pain as well as acupressure/acupuncture points. Magnets are safe as usually there is not much of a side effect, except that they should not be overused lest overstimulation at times leads to dizziness. As such magnets can be safely used for a short duration under the supervision of a Magnet Therapist.

Here we would like to provide some tips to be adopted in your life to be followed as a preventive measure:

Reduce the intake of salt since a high salt intake is considered to be a major causative factor for the onset of this condition as it causes loss of calcium through the kidneys.

Take up exercises, e.g. shoulder, hip and leg exercises, to keep yourself more active and self-sufficient and strengthening the muscles and bones, thereby reducing the risk of injuries.

Adopt exercises to strengthen your back muscles. Back bone is the region of concern as when the bones in this area of the body get weaker supported with weak muscles, the posture changes over the shoulders and the back. Studies have shown that with an increase in the strength in the back muscles, the risk factor of the fractures in the vertebral column is comparatively reduced. Pelvic tilt may be the starting point for strengthening your back muscles.

Lie on your back with knees bent. Place a pillow and a rolled towel under your head and neck respectively for support. Inhale allowing your chest and belly expand. Hold for some time. While exhaling, flatten your back into the floor by tightening your stomach muscles. Inhale deeply again and repeat the process of squeezing your abdominal muscles in the zone of your naval. This exercise has to be done only for a few minutes.

Importance of walking to overcome the incidence of bone loss needs no emphasis. Studies have shown that the people who walked for over 30 minutes a day experienced less deformity in the region of their spines when compared to their counterparts, who did not walk at all. Other studies have also shown that incidence of bone loss in those who walk regularly was comparatively much lesser than those in non-walkers. Walk could be brisk but no jogging, jumping or over-stressing your joints is permissible and, as such, needs to be avoided. The entire skeleton takes the load of your body weight and it results in strengthening of the muscles, our bone formation and also it helps strengthen our backbone. Pay attention that while walking, you breathe deep, walk straight and watch your steps.

To take care of diet part, for boosting/maintaining the calcium balance in your bones:

Take adequate quantity of yogurt or cottage cheese that boosts calcium in our bones.

Those who have allergy to milk or want to avoid milk, another way to get adequate calcium is to take juices fortified with calcium citrate.

Eat lot of green-leafy vegetables, broccoli, etc. They have plenty of calcium to supply to our body.

Magnesium is also supposed to influence our bone health. As such, try to get adequate quantity of it in the shape of consumption of legumes, vegetables and whole-grains.

Eggs too are good for our bones. As such, consume at least an egg every other day if not daily.

Likewise, manganese has to play an important role in taking care of osteoporsis. Try to ensure daily intake of this mineral to the extent of 2 to 5 mg. Pineapples, rice and almonds are rich source of this mineral besides whole-grains, nuts, green, leafy vegetables and tea, etc.

Spinach, kale, lettuce, avocados, and broccoli are rich in Vitamin K, which wards off hip fracture in case consumed in adequate quantity.

Mind the consumption of protein as too much of it could result into bone loss.

Vitamin C actually helps build the foundation that makes up bone structure. As such, include adequate supply of Vitamin C in your diet plan. Strawberries, mango, cantaloupe, kiwi fruit, water melon, etc. are rich sources of Vitamin C.

Including Omega 3 fatty acids is equally important, as they produce more bone proteins that provide the basis to the body to lay down minerals, e.g. calcium, phosphorus, and magnesium that help in building up the bone density, thereby reducing the risk of osteoporosis in our life. As such, consumption of the fish containing Omega 3 is beneficial as good fats contained in fish help us in maintaining the levels of cholesterol and triglyceride in check. It also helps in protecting us from blood clots.

Yet another product you can hardly afford to neglect, in case you are conscious of the health of your bones, are soya foods (TOFU). They are known to reduce cholesterol, mitigate the discomfort during menopause, maintain elasticity of blood vessels, preventing blood clotting to quite an extent as also try to help human body from fighting malignant tumors. They are known to contain 'isoflavones' in abundance, an element which is responsible for bone health to a great extent.

□

Case–45
Daily Workout Programme for Keeping Fit

Of late, we have observed that as and when a new patient is brought to our clinic, the attendant(s) accompanying the patient generally asks a question, out of curiosity, as to whether acupressure technique could also be adopted to keep fit, as also can it be practised as self-help by them as a daily work-out programme, i.e. as preventive medicine. Appreciating the concern of the people, in view of their growing awareness about the side effect of the medicine as also their desire and the amount of effort people have started laying over fitness, with a view to reach the stage when they have no other option but to take recourse to medication, we decided to incorporate the usage of acupressure technique as a self-help care programme. We have the satisfaction that innumerable number of people have benefitted after following the below-mentioned regime.

We strongly feel that in all fairness, we can adopt acupressure as a way of life to keep fit. All that is required is to follow a schedule of around 12 pressure points as discussed hereinafter. This way, we can say for sure that in case one adopts the routine of taking pressure over these pressure points daily for a period of seven days, to begin with, press them alternate days next two weeks and reduce it to pressing merely once a week, the incidence of falling sick shall be reduced substantially.

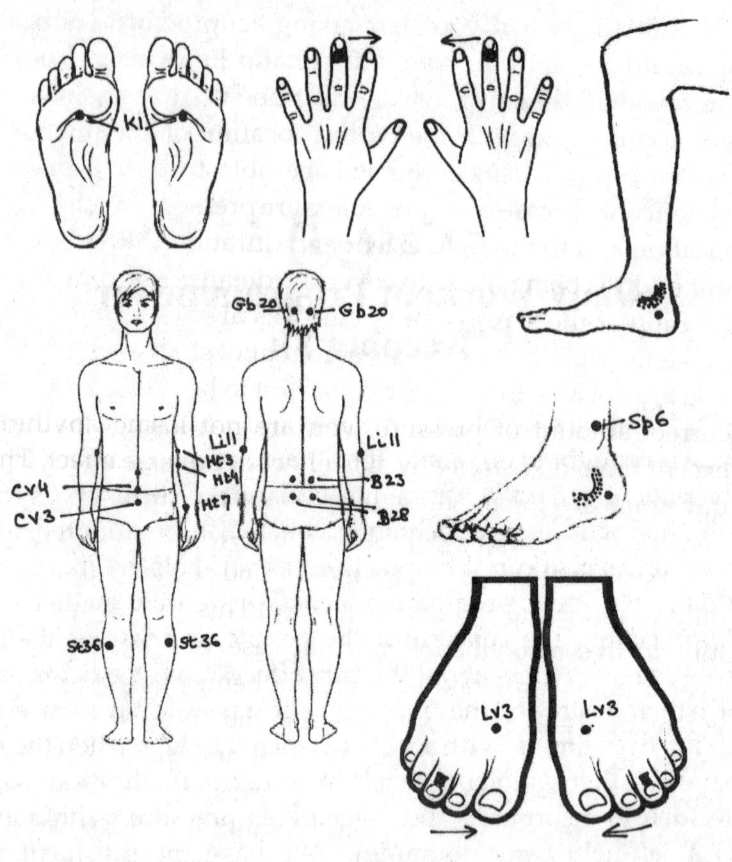

As a word of caution, here we would like to mention very clearly that adopting the abovesaid self-care measures are meant to inculcate amongst the masses awareness about health care as a preventive part only. In no way, these measures should be adopted in isolation in case onset of any major disease is even suspected. In such an eventuality, immediate medical advice from a professional practising conventional medicine should be sought. Under no circumstances, one should feel that this branch of Science is self-sufficient to take care of even ailments of even serious nature, which could lead to life-threatening condition.

Initially, when you start taking acupressure yourself, it would be better to have a first-hand knowledge from a professional therapist, maybe just one or two sessions, to get acclimatised with the correct location of the intended pressure points, since you will be able to derive proper benefit only in case pressure points are pressed over the right location and to the right extent and duration. Although all-out effort is being made to cover the details regarding exact location of those pressure points, it is always important to make the right beginning. Be sure that even in case initially you are not able to reach the right spot to be pressed, or take correct amount of pressure, you are not losing anything except time, no fear of any side effect or adverse effect. The day you learn to take pressure over the right spot in a right manner to the right extent, it is a win-win situation. Each point can be pressed for up to 30 to 60 seconds, applying mild to moderate, yet firm, pressure. This too should be in four to five installments. Since in case you give pressure over a point for a minute, the area being touched might get tender, and when you press it the next day, it may hurt you over that location. You will notice that once you have learnt the correct location of a pressure point, as well as an idea of how much pressure could be given without creating tenderness, you will be able to complete the work out programme in a maximum period of 20 minutes or so. One more thing we would like to clarify in this regard, to make the concept clearer, is that there is no hard and fast rule about the chronological order in which these pressure points need to be pressed. You may go according to your convenience, applying pressure over the pressure point that you can access easily.

To begin with, take pressure over Li-4, as shown in the diagram. This point is located at the crease that is formed when we join the thumb and the index finger. It is known by the name 'Adjoining Valley'. This point is considered to be a very important pressure point as it is capable of relaxing the muscles, balance the flow of energy in the upper and lower part of the body. It also activates the bowel movement besides its usefulness in relieving headache and pain in other parts of the body, since body tends to release natural pain-killers, known as endorphins, when this point is stimulated. Since this point is also used for inducing labor, pregnant women should refrain from pressing this point for uterine constrictions may be caused.

Next, we can apply pressure over Li 11, known by the name 'Pool at the Crook'. It is located at the outer end of the crease that is formed when we bend our hand and touch our shoulder. Since this point gets very tender to touch, pressure needs to be given with utmost care, even by rubbing over the area. An extremely useful point for clearing excess heat and dampness from the body, as also pain in elbow, arm and stiffness/pain in the shoulder area. It has been found to be a very potent point in healing 'tennis elbow', as also 'allergies', asthma, etc.

Further to the above, St-36 and Sp-6 need to be pressed. Whereas St-36 is located four-finger width below the patellar bone (knee cap). Pressed in combination with Sp-6, we are able to tonify Ch'i and improve blood flow to bring vitality. This point is known as 'Three Mile Foot' also. It has also been found to be having a positive stimulative effect over the stomach meridian. Sp-6 is known by the name 'Three Yin Meeting Point'. As its very name suggests, it strengthens the 'Yin' of three meridians at the same time, viz. kidney, liver, and spleen. This point is considered to be master point for overcoming any sort of female problems, e.g. regulating periods, relieving cramps, facilitating menopause. This vital point is located above the ankle bone towards the inside of the leg on the back side, i.e. achilles tendon.

Hereinafter, pressure can be given over the point Lv-3 (Bigger Rushing), is located at two-finger-width above the web between the big toe and the second toe. As this point also tends to get very tender soon, we should start giving only 'mild' pressure over this point, to begin with and then gradually switch over to 'moderate' pressure. Giving pressure over this point on both the feet simultaneously has been found to be all the more beneficial. This point is known for its capability to boost immunity in our body.

This may be followed by giving pressure over the back edge of the ankle bone and the achilles tendon, as shown in the figure. This point is known as Kd 3 (Supreme Stream). Known as the root of the Yin and Yang of our entire body. It is considered to be the prime source point in respect of the kidney meridian. It is also known for its powerful tonifying effect on the entire body.

After giving pressure as above, press B-23, which is located 1-1/2 inches over either side of the spine, above the level of your naval and below the centre of the back, as shown in the figure. Both these points can also be stimulated with your fists rubbing over that area. Stimulating this point in association with Kd-3 tonifies Ch'i of the kidney meridian in a big way.

Hereinafter, give pressure over Gb 20 (Wind Pool), located in the depression on either side of the spine over your neck, one thumb-width above the hairline, at the base of the skull. Over this point, pressure could be given with the help of both of your thumbs simultaneously. It helps in alleviating the stiffness in the neck area, headache, pain in shoulders, etc. It also regulates the internal movement of energy in our body.

To stop stagnation of blood in the lower abdominal area as also for nourishing effect in our skin, press Sp-10 (Sea of Blood). This point is located two-thumb-width above the knee over the bulge of the thigh muscle towards the interior side.

Pressure over St-40, a point located half-way between the ankle bone on the outside of the foot and centre of knee cap, over the tibia and go two-thumb-width of the bone on the outside. This point is highly beneficial in eliminating mucus and congestion.

To conclude, give pressure over the extra points as shown in the figure. These points lie over the middle of the right as well as left forearms. Whereas the point over the right hand lies half-way between the right elbow and the crease over the wrist. It helps prevent the loss of energy from our body, the pressure point over the same location on the left forearm a thumb width of the bone to the outside, known as Pc 4, is known to stimulate the heart.

This regime of 12 master points can be adopted as your way of life, along with the routine of exercising or diet programme you may be following to attain a state of well being and fitness.

□

Case–46
Immunity

Our immune system is a complex network that involves our entire body. Each one of them has been assigned a role to play in reinforcing our defence against outside attack, maybe some virus or otherwise. To elaborate a bit, skin is the first line of defence against the viruses. Lymph glands produce and store numerous white blood cells to provide protection to our body from disease. Our thoughts, positive or negative, leave a vital impact over our immunity. Our immune system is so designed that it locates and destroys bacteria the moment they enter our system. Energy imbalances also weaken our immune system. It has been established beyond doubt that stress in any form may be excesses we do in our day-to-day life, such as excess of any activity like lying down; stress over our eyes or even emotional stress; physical exertion; sitting or standing might be causing some damage to our body. Large intestines and lung meridian are adversely affected in case we keep lying all the time. Putting excessive strain over our eyes or emotional stress may cause adverse impact on heart and small intestines. Gallbladder and liver are affected by excessive physical exertion. Those who keep sitting might feel the impact in the shape of adverse reaction from their stomach and spleen meridians and damage may be caused in case of those who keep standing and may be exhibited in the shape of fatigue/backaches.

As such, in our day-to-day conduct, whereas on one hand, we should be conscious that we do not expose

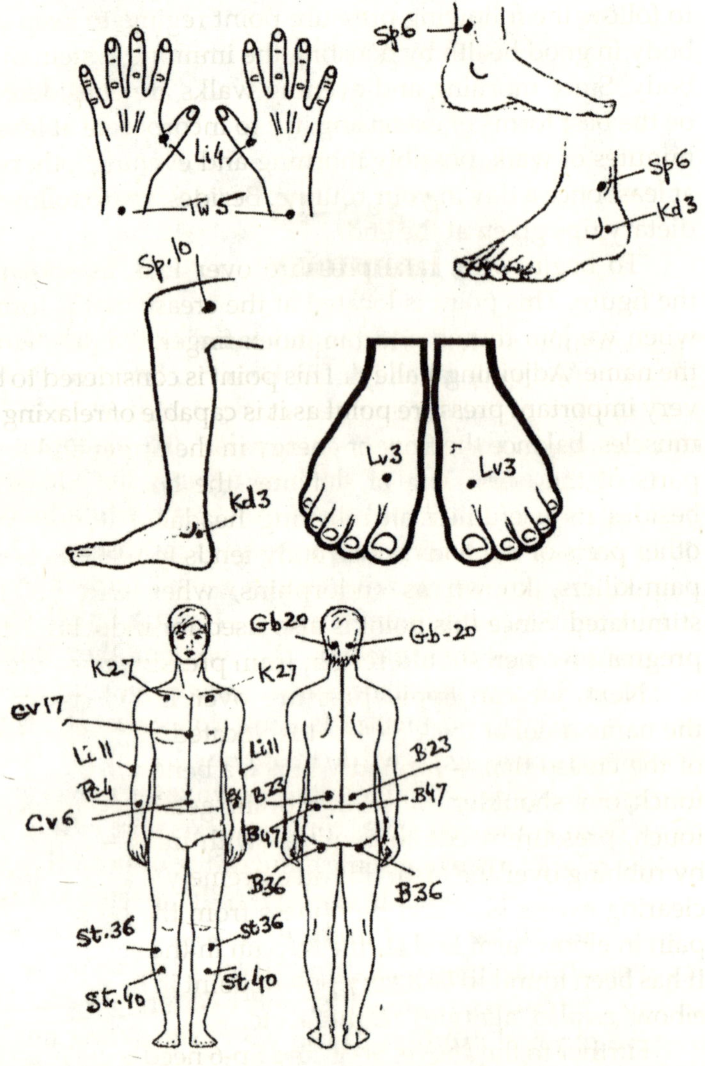

our body to undue stress under any circumstances. On the other hand, we pay adequate attention towards our lifestyle by adopting yoga, breathing exercises and dietary modifications in our life from time to time, with a view to increase our energy level as also immune system. Also try to follow the following pressure point regime to keep your body in good health by boosting the immune system in our body. Since morning and evening walks are considered to be the best forms of exercising, try to incorporate at least 30 minutes of walk, possibly morning and evening, otherwise at least once a day in your routine. Besides, try to follow the dietary tips given at the end.

To begin with, take pressure over Li-4, as shown in the figure. This point is located at the crease that is formed when we join thumb and the index finger. It is known by the name 'Adjoining Valley'. This point is considered to be a very important pressure point as it is capable of relaxing the muscles, balance the flow of energy in the upper and lower parts of the body. It also activates the bowel movement besides its usefulness in relieving headache and pain in other parts of the body, since body tends to release natural pain-killers, known as endorphins, when this point is stimulated. Since this point is also used for inducing labor, pregnant women should refrain from pressing this point.

Next, we can apply pressure over Li-11, known by the name 'Pool at the Crook'. It is located at the outer end of the crease that is formed when we bend our hand and touch our shoulder. Since this point gets very tender to touch, pressure needs to be given with utmost care, even by rubbing over the area. It is an extremely useful point for clearing excess heat and dampness from the body, as also pain in elbow, arm and stiffness/pain in the shoulder area. It has been found to be a very potent point in healing 'tennis elbow' as also 'allergies', asthma, etc.

Further to the above, St-36 and Sp-6 need to be pressed. Whereas St-36 is located four-finger width below the patellar bone (knee cap). Pressed in combination with Sp-6, we are able to tonify Ch'i and improve blood flow to bring vitality. This point is known as 'Three Mile Foot' also. It has also been found to be having a positive stimulative effect over the stomach meridian. Sp-6 is known by the name 'Three

Yin Meeting Point'. As its very name suggests, it strengthens the 'Yin' of three meridians at the same time, viz. kidney, liver, and spleen. This point is considered to be master point for overcoming any sort of female problems, e.g. regulating periods, relieving cramps, facilitating menopause. This vital point is located above the ankle bone towards the inside of the leg on the back side, i.e. achilles tendon.

Hereinafter, pressure can be given over the point Lv-3 (Bigger Rushing), is located at two-finger-width above the web between the big toe and the second toe. As this point also tends to get very tender soon, we should start giving only 'mild' pressure over this point, to begin with and then gradually switch over to 'moderate' pressure. Giving pressure over this point on both the feet simultaneously has been found to be all the more beneficial. This point is known for its capability to boost immunity in our body.

This may be followed by giving pressure over the back edge of the ankle bone and the achilles tendon, as shown in the figure. This point is known as Kd-3 (Supreme Stream). Known as the root of the Yin and Yang of our entire body. Is considered to be the prime source point in respect of the kidney meridian. It is also known for its powerful tonifying effect on the entire body.

After giving pressure as above, press B-23, which is located 1-1/2 inches over either side of the spine, above the level of your naval and below the centre of the back, as shown in the figure. Both these points can also be stimulated with your fists rubbing over that area. Stimulating this point in association with Kds-3 tonifies Ch'i of the kidney meridian in a big way.

Hereinafter, give pressure over Gb-20 (wind pool), located in the depression on either side of the spine over your neck, one thumb-width above the hairline, at the base of the skull. Over this point, pressure could be given with the help of both of your thumbs simultaneously. It helps in alleviating the stiffness in the neck area, headache, pain in shoulders, etc. It also regulates the internal movement of energy in our body.

To stop stagnation of blood in the lower abdominal area as also for nourishing effect in our skin, press Sp-10 (Sea of Blood). This point is located two-thumb-width above the knee over the bulge of the thigh muscle towards the interior side.

Pressed over St-40, a point located half-way between the ankle bone on the outside of the foot and centre of knee cap, over the tibia and go two-thumb-width of the bone on the outside. This point is highly beneficial in eliminating mucus and congestion.

B-36, named Bearing Support, is known for providing the power of resistance to our body, specially from cold and flu. It is said that cold and wind enters from the skin from this point. As such, giving pressure over this area shall provide the body power to overcome the intrusion of Flu and cold. This point is located over the hip bone, as shown in the figure.

Similarly, giving pressure over the pressure point known by the name Elegant Mansion (K-27), which lies in the depression below the clavical bone, as shown in the figure, has been found to be very useful in stimulating the immune system as it helps combat and relieve breathing problems, ease chest congestion, coughing in the asthmatic patients and, to a great extent, patients suffering from high level of anxiety or suffering from depression.

Yet another pressure point that needs to be pressed in the cycle is Cv-6 (known as Sea of Energy). As its name itself suggests, it strengthens the immune system as also internal organs in our body. It has also been found to be very useful in alleviating general weakness, gastric problem, Constipation, pain in the abdomen besides being highly beneficial in overcoming female problems by stimulating the reproductive system. This point is located two-finger-widths below the belly button, above the pubic bone.

Pressure over this area can be given by rubbing that area gently, with three fingers joined together at an angle of 30 to 45 degrees, as this area is a bit tender. Duration could be upto 30 seconds.

Tw-5, known by the name outer gate, is located about two-finger-width above the back of the middle of the wrist crease, between the ulna and radius bones in the forearm. This pressure point is known to improve the resistance power of the body besides being beneficial in alleviating wrist pain, heel pain, rheumatism, and tendonitis.

Yet another point that re-inforces the immune system is named Sea of Vitality, B-47, is located in the lower back four-finger-width away from the vertebrae column, at waist level. This point is known for overcoming fatigue and lower back pain.

Cv-17, called Sea of Tranquility, is known for its power to boost immune system as also improving the functioning of thymus gland. It also helps reducing anxiety levels and depression, etc. It is located over the centre of the breast bone-three-thumb width above the base of the sternum bone, almost at the level a line drawn from the nipples of the breasts would intersect.

To conclude, give pressure over the extra points as shown in the figures. These points lie over the middle of the right as well as left forearms. Whereas the point over the right hand lies half-way between the right elbow and the crease over the wrist. It helps prevent the loss of energy from our body, the pressure point over the same location on the left forearm a thumb width of the bone to the outside , known as Pc-4, is known to Stimulate the Heart.

This regime of the points discussed above can be adopted as a part of your plan to boost the immunity of a patient who may be bed ridden and may be suffering from some terminal disease of the sort of even cancer, as while undergoing chemotherapy, etc., the immunity of the body is almost lost. Giving pressure over these points has been found to be of a substantial relief. Care has, however, to be taken that whereas it is important to give pressure over all the pressure points discussed above, it may not be possible to or, in the interest of the patient, to handle so many points at a time, as such the plan should be drawn in such a manner that almost all the pressure points are pressed at least three to four times a week to get better results.

As for the people who want to boost their immunity as a preventive, the above schedule of pressure points can be adopted for a week, all points in one session, thereafter choosing some points on a particular day and next set of points the other day. Besides, they may continue with their routine of exercising or diet programme they may be following, to attain a state of well-being and fitness.

Adopting the usage of soy, fresh vegetables, mildly roasted sesame seeds, beans, salads, and soups would help strengthen the immune system, thereby enhancing the body's ability to protect itself from disease. We should try avoid taking canned and processed food, as their food value is lost in the process of processing.

Likewise, try to focus on deep breathing, trying to breathe deep, each breath deeper than the previous one. Inhale and exhale smoothly, letting your body relax, try to feel the breath vitalising your body.

□

Case–47
Low Back Pain/Incontinence/Prostate

I recall of an old patient of mine Mr. W, around 79 years of age from Gurgaon. He was suffering from lower back, hip pain, prostate, and incontinence for almost six to seven years. Looking into his age, he was not desirous of undergoing surgery. On the recommendation of an old patient of mine, he agreed to take treatment from me. This was in the year 2001, in case I can properly recall. He told me that he had to get up upto four times in the night to pass urine. Although he feels lot of pressure over the bladder as if he will pass urine in the bed itself, but since he had pain in the lower back too, which he said radiates downwards upto the calf muscle (a sign of sciatica pain) and that he might not be able to move fast at the last minute, fearing that he might not spoil the bed, he makes a move towards the toilet in anticipation. Despite lot of pressure and urge to urinate, he shared that it takes time in starting to void himself. At times, he informed that despite his going to void himself a number of times, when he feels that he has passed urine fully, he complained that he spoils his trousers as urine dribbles out at the end, also complained of burning sensation during or after passing urine, an indication enough to define the status of his prostate gland.

The first day when he visited my clinic, he took approximately four minutes' time to cover the distance of about 20-25 feet from where he had to get down from car

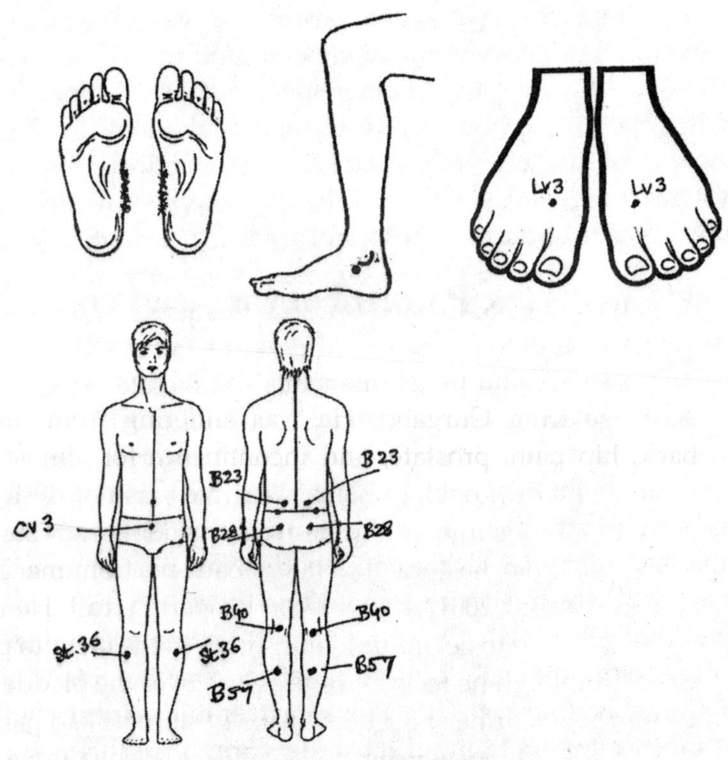

and entering the clinic area, that too with the help of a stick he had to use for support while walking.

These conditions are enough to establish the onset of the disease, which is generally confined to inflammation of the prostate. It would be wise to get yourself examined by your family physician, in case you feel that you have even some of the aforesaid symptoms, with a view to rule out the probability of malignancy, before going in for any sort of treatment the non-conventional way. Time and again, we have been stressing the need for co-management of case(s) of this nature and the results have been quite encouraging. In the instant case, Mr. W confirmed that he had undergone physical examination and all the requisite tests to rule out any sort of malignancy.

To begin with, started giving pressure over LV-3 point. This point lies between the big and second toe, about two finger width above Lv-2 point, which lies at the junction of the big and second toe, on the top of the foot. Lv-3 is known for its tonifying effect over the entire immune system. It regulates the Ch'i in the liver meridian which is considered to be the most powerful organ for 'detoxification' Thereafter, pressed Sp-6, the three meeting point, which is located above the ankle bone towards the inside of the leg on the back side, four finger width above the ankle bone, a highly potent point to simultaneously stimulate kidneys, liver and spleen meridians and is considered to be very important for providing relief in the instant condition. In continuity with this point, pressure was given at St-36. This pressure point strengthens the entire body, tones up the muscles and revitalises the entire body. Next point pressed was Cv-3, which is located about one-thumb-width below Cv-4 (known as Gate Origin), which is located four finger width below the belly button. Its effect over the 'bladder meridian' is almost specific. Pressure over this point should be given after emptying the bladder. Stimulate this point for about a minute, gently. This can be followed by giving pressure at B-28, which is an associated point for urinary bladder, located at about one-and-a-half inches on either side of the spine as shown in the figure. Thereafter give pressure on B-23, located in the middle of the waist, almost half-way between the rib cage and the hipbone as shown in the figure. This point is known for its effect on sex organs and, as a result, helps in overcoming prostate problem. Also gave pressure around the ankles of both the feet on both anterior and posterior sides as shown by the dotted lines in the figure as also over the mid-point between the lowest portion of the ankle and the heel (diagonally) as shown in the figure. Followed by giving rolling pressure over the reflex area relating to the urinary bladder which lies in the lumbosacral part of the spine with a view to strengthen the urinary bladder.

Thereafter, with a view to provide him a bit of immediate relief, gave pressure over both soles using 'thumb walk' technique for about 2-3 minutes, followed by giving massage-like pressure over the achilles tendon area (the area behind the leg above the heel). This is the area from where the sciatic nerve passes behind the ankles and goes down to the bottom of the heels, on both anterior and posterior sides of the heel. This was followed by giving pressure over the 'lumbosacral' area of the vertebral column, marked as 'XXXXX' in the figure. This was done keeping in mind the fact that often sciatic pain is caused by the rupture or a slip-disc in the lower lumbar area. Points indicated are the pressure points where the sciatic nerve ends over the heel. Point shown on the back of the heel is the point B-28 which pertains to the area falling over the hip joint area. This point hurts a lot on being pressed but has been found to be extremely beneficial in overcoming any sort of discomfort in the lower back area.

This was followed by giving pressure over B-40 (middle of the Crooke), which is located in the middle of the back of your knee, in the centre between the two tendons over the crease formed when you bend your knee. This point is also known by the name 'Command Point' for its powerful influence on the lower back problems. Then gave pressure on B-23 point, as shown in the figure. This point has been found to be of immense help in alleviating lower back pain, sciatica and fatigue caused due to severe pain in that area. This was followed by giving pressure over B-47, as shown. This point when pressed in conjunction with B-23 helps a lot in providing relief in the pain in the lower back region besides helping in overcoming fatigue, besides calming down the irritated sciatic nerve. Further to this, i pressed B-48, which helps provide relief in sciatica, hip pain, lower back pain and in alleviating tension in the region.

Next day when Mr. W came for the session, he was happy to inform that the previous night he had to get up only two times to go to the toilet. Also reported that he felt a bit of relief in the intensity of pain in the lower back, though he said the pain returned after some time. This was not a news to me, as most of the patients, when they come back the next day, report of some relief for a short time only and report that the pain came back. However, we consider it as a signal from the patient towards body response, as we call it. It is a sort of indicator that the body responded. Next two days, Mr. W had nothing further to report. The fourth day when he came, he was too excited and informed by raising both his hands in the air, that doctor today it took me only two minutes to cover the distance of 20-25 feet from the car to your clinic and that he has been able to walk without any support from the stick.

In all, it took around 14 sessions to get almost total recovery. By this time, Mr. W had recovered almost 85%. Generally, I ask my patients to stop coming to me once they attain recovery to the extent of 80% or above, as rest of the recovery comes on its own. Moreover at the age of 79 years, perhaps we cannot aspire for a 100% recovery and that too without any sort of medication.

□

Case–48

Heart Attack/Hypotension/ Stoppage of Urine

I recall of a very old case somewhere in the year 1998-99. I was informed that one of our relations, Mr. L, aged about 70 years, was critically ill and had to be admitted to a private nursing home in Meerut. Much details were not available about the nature of the condition of the patient except that he had suffered some heart problem. Some outsider had simply informed about the admission of the patient with the request to try and reach Meerut at the earliest. As I had some compulsions in Delhi, I could not go there immediately and reached after around 10 hours of the episode. Meanwhile, the other member of the family, who had reached there much earlier, informed that Mr. L had suffered a heart attack and according to the doctors attending him, certain complications had developed and they had informed the family that his condition was critical and, that is why, he was kept in CCU.

When I reached the hospital, I was informed that though the attack was not a major one, yet since the blood pressure had dipped to 78/45 and to add to it, the patient was not in a position to pass urine. The doctors were unable to put him on diuretics in the wake of such low blood pressure. They had asked the family member to wait and watch and that they were taking every possible action to save the life.

When I saw the patient and the reports, etc., I found that perhaps there was not much of an imminent risk to life

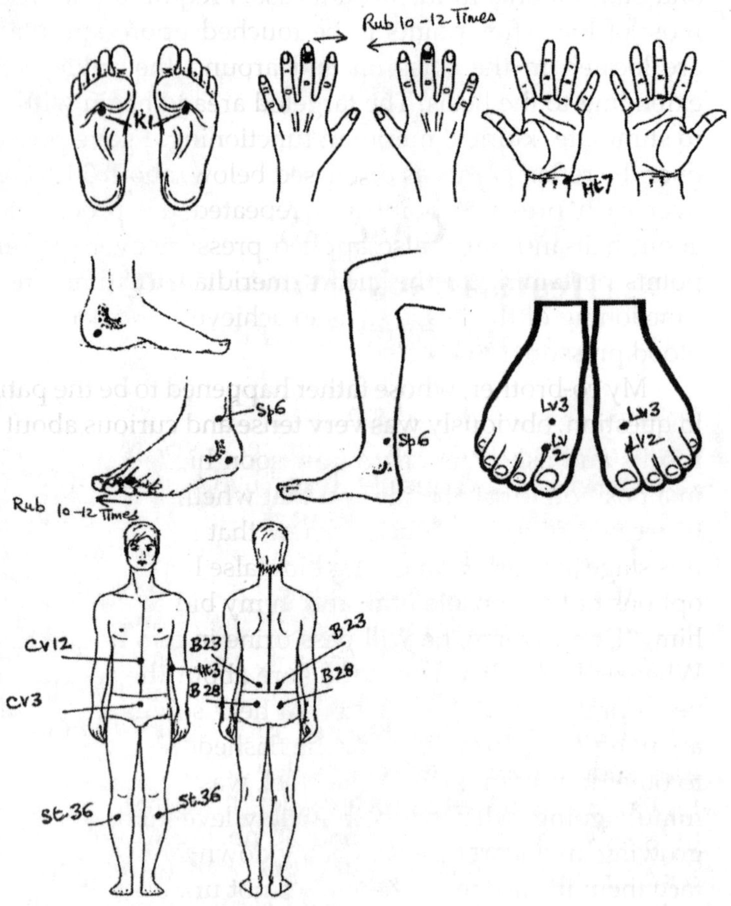

in case somehow the patient could be made to pass urine in a natural way. As such, introduced myself to the attending cardiologist, sought his permission to give pressure over certain points over and around the heels of the feet to try to facilitate urination. Initially, the doctor was apprehensive as to how this could be possible, yet somehow I was permitted to touch the patient's feet, and that is what I required, as administration of 'acupressure technique', to drive benefit by making the various systems in our body work in a particular way, is possible by giving pressure over soles and palms alone. In the instant case, I required only feet as most of the reflex points to be touched upon (stimulated) are located in the soles on and around the ankle bones, extending to the heels. The targeted area to begin with was to stimulate 'kidney' meridian functioning. I gave pressure over the reflex points as discussed below, about 30 seconds over each pressure point and repeated the process after about half-an-hour. I also applied pressure over the reflex points pertaining to the 'heart' meridian to stimulate the functioning of the heart, so as to achieve some boost in the blood pressure too.

My co-brother, whose father happened to be the patient in question, obviously was very tense and curious about the results and asked me as to how soon his father would be in a position to pass urine and that whether he will be able to recover from the attack. I knew that saying anything at this stage amounted to giving him false hopes. Yet I had no options but to console him, and in my bid to do that, I told him, "Don't worry, he will pass urine in two hours' time." Whereas I myself was not too sure about the results to be very frank. He was so excited to hear something positive about his father recovery, that he flashed the probable news to other family members. The clock was ticking with every minute going, whereas their anxiety level and hopes were growing, my heart beat was going down, as to how I would face them in case the patient does not urinate in two hours told by me. I had obtained very good results from these pressure points in the past too, but the patients were certainly not in such a critical condition. Anyway, as they say, the time goes on, it went on and ultimately the prayers of all the relations around and the miracle of the pressure point technique applied yielded result and in exactly one hour and 50 minutes' time from the moment pressure was given to him, the patient passed about 20 ml of urine. Encouraged by the results, the doctors attending him allowed me to co-manage the patient and I started giving him pressure regularly, two times a day till he was in the hospital for the next three days, when he was discharged. The following regime of pressure point schedule was followed:

To begin with, I started giving pressure over Lv-3 point. This point lies between the big and second toe, about two finger width above Lv-2 point, which lies at the junction of the big and second toe, on the top of the foot. Lv-3 is known for its tonifying effect over the entire immune system. It regulates the Ch'i in the liver meridian which is considered to be the most powerful organ for 'detoxification'. Thereafter, pressed Sp-6, the three meeting point, which is located above the ankle bone towards the inside of the leg on the back side, four finger width above the ankle bone, a highly potent point to simultaneously stimulate kidneys, liver and spleen meridians and is considered to be very important for providing relief in the instant condition. In continuity with this point pressure should be given at St.-36, this pressure point strengthens the entire body, tones up the muscles and revitalizes the entire body. Next point pressed was Cv-3, which is located about one thumb width below Cv-4 (known as Gate Origin) which is located four finger widths below the belly button. Its effect over the 'bladder meridian' is almost specific. Pressure over this point should be given after emptying the bladder. Stimulate this point for a few minutes, gently. This can be followed by giving pressure at B-28, which is an associated point for urinary bladder, located at about one and a half inches on either side of the spine as shown in the figure. Thereafter give pressure on B-23, located in the middle of the waist, almost halfway between the rib cage and the hip bone as shown. This point is known for its effect on sexual reproductivity organs and as a result helps in over coming Prostate problem. Giving final touches to the session, gave pressure around the ankles of both the feet on both anterior and posterior sides as shown by the dotted lines in the figure as also over the midpoint between the lowest portion of the ankle and the heel (diagonally). Followed by giving rolling pressure over the reflex area relating to the urinary bladder which lies in the lumbo sacral part of the spine with a view to strengthen the gave pressure over Lv-3 point which lies between the big and the second toe on top of the foot. This point tonifies the liver and the flow of Ch'i in the liver meridian, as one of the prominent causes of hypotension is blockage in the liver meridian and stimulating this point removes stagnation/ blockage. This was followed by giving pressure over Lv-2. This point lies at the junction of the big toe and the second toe. Is known by the name 'Xingjian' and is known to stimulate 'Yin' and Sedate 'Yang' of liver, when pressed in combination with Lv-3. Also pressed Cv-12, which is located along the midline of the abdomen, a little above the umbilicum and is considered to be almost a specific point to control hypotension.

Then gave pressure over Ht-7 as well as Ht-3 on the little finger side, precisely about two finger widths below the elbow joint. Ht-7 lies just at the crease where the lower arm and the palm meet towards the little finger side. Giving pressure in the area, where the nail ends and the thin skin begins, over the middle finger, in the indicated direction over both feet and the hands has been found to be very effective in controlling low blood pressure.

Also gave pressure over K-1 point, which is located in the depression appearing on the sole of the foot when the foot is in plantar flexion, at the junction of the anterior and middle third of the sole approximately. This pressure point is considered to be a highly potent revival point as also known for being highly beneficial in stimulating the heart. □

Case–49
Meniere's Disease

About six years ago, in the year 2010, a case was brought to my clinic, the patient Mrs. M was 56 years of age and had been suffering from Meniere's disease for more than six to seven years. She had undergone treatment under almost every stream of medicine. She reported that every time she switched on to a different stream of treatment, she became hopeful as it showed some positive results, but soon, say within a day or two or so, her symptoms of tinnitus, deafness and vertigo started showing up again. She had become so frustrated that when she was brought to me, she told me at the outset that I will try your therapy only for four days and shall discontinue in case I do not see any signs of recovery. I tried to bring round the point to her that in the stream of science, I deal with, there shall be no medication, whereas thus far, she had been getting drugs, anti-depressants as well as even tranquillizers, as such it would not be in the overall interest in case we commence the treatment on a conditional basis. At last, she agreed to take treatment for a week and then decide what to do. Besides above, the patient presented other symptoms, e.g. dizziness, ringing in the ears as well as blocked sinuses also.

It may be pertinent to mention here that these days more and more patients suffering from this condition are reporting. One of the probable causes might be frequent usage of blood thinners to ward of cardiac and neurological problems, or to combat arthritic conditions or young boys and girls working in call centers or others using headphones

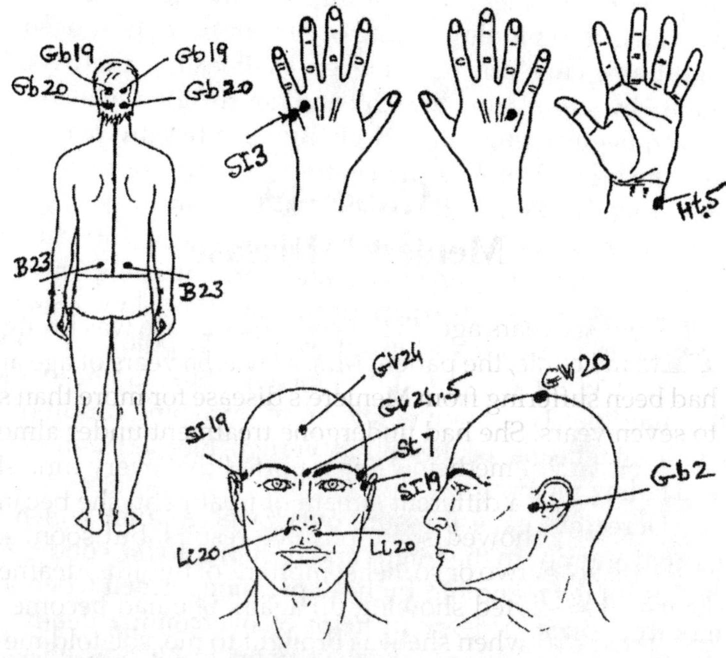

or remaining glued to cell phones for hours at a stretch. Investigations, e.g. MRI, eudiometry, balance tests, and X-ray cervical spine did not indicate any major problem except that the patient had undergone noticeable hearing loss, yet the patient had severe symptoms. She complained of occassional sleeplessness (insomnia) and vertigo. Yet another condition she presented was acute sinusitis, which according to her had been causing her lots of restlessness. Here for the benefit of the readers, it may be mentioned that sinuses are the empty spaces in the bones of the skull, normally filled with air. Inflammation of the sinuses with excessive formation of secretions from its linings, which might get infected is called 'sinusitis'.

Another feature presented by this patient was dizziness, the causative factors could be menopause, motion sickness or migraine. In these conditions, the patient feels light-headedness, or the feeling of spinning is presented. Some infection or imbalance in the fluids in the inner ear could also cause the spinning feeling or dizziness. In most of such conditions, cure can be achieved by boosting the overall vitality by stimulating the Ch'i and nourishing the blood.

To begin with, I started giving her pressure over Gv-20, which is located in the centre of the top of our skull. The exact location of this point can be seen in the figure. This point is very helpful in aleviating discomfort due to dizziness, insomnia, memory, and concentration, ringing in the ears, nasal obstruction and boosting low energy. Thereafter, pressure was given over Gv-24 point, which is located over the midline at the junction of the forehead and the hairline. This point is known to overcome conditions, e.g. frontal headache, insomnia, vertigo, blocked sinuses as also failing memory.

Hereafter, gave pressure over Si-19, a point which is located anterior to the tragus and posterior to the condyloid process of the mandible, in the depression formed when the mouth is open. This point helps in overcoming deafness, tinnitus, ear infection, etc. Next point to be pressed was Gb-2. This point too is very effective in getting relief from Deafness, tinnitus and toothaches, etc., besides being helpful in overcoming TMJ pain and facial paralysis and is located anterior to the intertragic notch as shown in the figure. St-7 was the next point to be pressed. This point too takes good care of deafness, tinnitus, ear infection, TMJ pain, etc. and is located at the lower border of the zygomatic arch, as has been indicated in the figure.

Next to this, went to press Li-20. This point is located at the mid-point of the lateral border of the nostril and has been found to be very useful in opening blockages of the maxillary sinuses, sinus headaches, nasal blockages as also as a facelift point. Hereafter, gave pressure over Tw-5. This point is located three finger breadths above the wrist crease on the dorsal side. It has been found to be very much beneficial in overcoming pain in the jaws, TMJ problems, deafness, ringing in the ears, sensation of plugged ears, as also to regulate abnormal heat sensation. Ht-5 was the next point to be pressed in the series. This point has tremendous healing effect on palpitation, dizziness, nervousness as well as pain in the wrist and the arm and is located one inch above the wrist crease on the ulnar side.

Further, to overcome ringing in the ears, headache, intracranial pressure increase, etc. pressed Si-3. This point is located, as shown in the figure, when a loose fist is made, it falls under the 5th metacarpal bone on the ulnar side. Gb-19 was the next point to be pressed. This point is located just above Gb-20 point, on the lateral side of the external occipital protuberance. It is very useful in conditions, e.g. headache, vertigo, tinnitus, wry neck and fits. With a view to boost energy, overcome deafness and ringing in the ears, pressure was given over Ub-23 point. This point is also known to overcome a number of male and female problems as also weakness of the knees and blurred vision. It is located three finger widths lateral to the lower border of the spine at second lumbar vertebra.

Till third session, the patient did not report even an iota of a change in her condition. However, when she turned up for the 4th session, she presented herself with a bit of smile over her face and told me that she has noticed some downfall in the intensity of the ringing of the bells in her ear as well as vertigo since the previous night. On my telling her that now onwards she can visit me every alternate day, she insisted that she would prefer to come everyday so that the relief attained is not lost. Even my trying to convince her that nothing of that sort should happen once relief starts, she insisted on visit on daily basis. After 8th session, she shared with me that she cannot recall that when in the past few years, she felt that feeling of wellness as she has been having for the last 24 hours. In all I gave her 15 sessions and she parted on a happy note, seeking excuses over her attitude and behaviour on telling me that she will try the acupressure therapy just for four days.

□

Case–50
Plantar Fasciitis/Excruciating Low Back Pain

Recently, while on a visit to the United States, I was introduced to a lady Ms. S, about 47 years of age. I was told that this female, who had been very friendly and helpful to everyone in the community, had been suffering for almost more than seven years in pain. I enquired in case she had any faith in non-conventional therapies, to which she replied that Sir, I am willing to undergo treatment under any therapy, all I aspire for is that I should get relief so that I may resume my active life once again and start helping the people around and get back to my exercises, as she was almost addicted to it. On asking what the problem was, she narrated that her disease has been diagnosed as 'plantar fascitis'. She further amplified saying that she finds it extremely difficult to walk as the heel of her right foot hurts like her feet is being pierced with a spear. Besides, she told that she feels pain in her lower back pointing towards her lumbosacral area. On further probing, she informed that the pain radiates down the right thigh up to the knee and, at times, even goes further down till the calf muscle.

It is the most common cause of inferior heel pain in the runners. Pain is more while rising up after prolonged sitting or early in the morning. The intensity of the pain and stiffness is reduced with activity but again returns after prolonged activity/standing. Maximum pain is felt on the

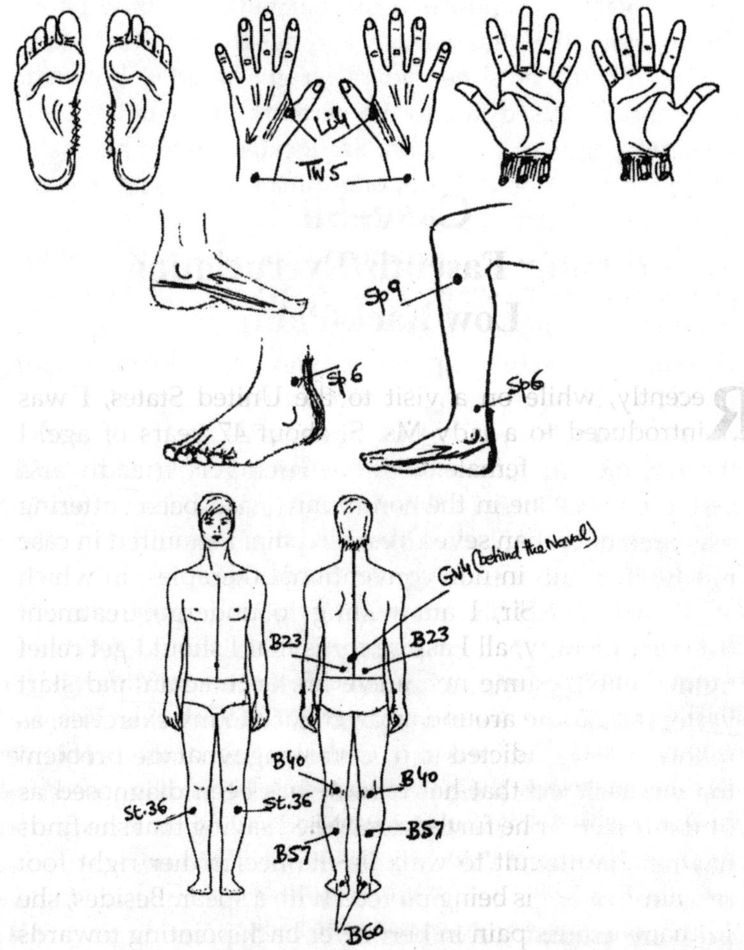

medial aspect of the calcaneus at the insertion of plantar fascia. Heel is one of the most important areas of our body as all six main meridians traverse the pelvic section of the heel. As a result, so many congestions can be traced to the meridians and their corresponding organs. The sciatic nerves are the largest nerves in our body connected to the lumbosacral area in the body. It passes through the buttocks down the back of the thighs and divides just above the knee joint into two branches known as tibial and peroneal nerves. Sciatica is indicated by sharp and stabbing pain in the leg along the sciatic nerve, at times from buttocks to the ankles. It could be either side, i.e. right or left or both sides even and is caused due to the vertebra pressing the nerve. The end-points of this nerve are located on the heel (soles of the foot), in a band about one-third way down the pad of the heel extending across the floor.

Looking into her condition as she was in tremendous pain despite being given a very heavy dose of pain-killers (800 mg of Ibufren twice a day), I decided to give her pressure by touching upon the reflex areas directly as also giving her pressure using 'acupressure technique' following the meridian theory. Further, she was advised to minimise the use of pain-killers to the extent possible and should take a pain-killer only when it was inescapable. Since she was tired of taking pain-killers and that too without getting much relief, she readily agreed for this too.

I commenced her treatment by giving pressure around the arch of the foot, over the area marked 'XXXX' in the figure, with a view to stimulate the lumbosacral part of the vertebral column, for about a minute on each side. This was followed by giving pressure as shown, the shaded area over the wrist of both hands on both sides by giving pressure in the direction indicated with the help of an arrow, after having stimulated this area for about a minute or so, gave pressure over points marked 1 to 6. Thereafter, I gave pressure around the ankles of both the feet, in particular over the affected feet, around the dotted lines as shown in the figure. Pressure was also given over Achilles tendon area shown with the help of dotted lines. I also gave pressure over the area depicted by the dotted lines in figures over the back of the palms and the anterior side of the feet, in the indicated direction. It has been observed that giving pressure over these areas which has a direct impact over the nervous system, provides much relief to the patients suffering from heel pain.

This was followed by giving pressure over Tw-5 point (at times, massage-like pressure has to be given over this point as it gets tender very soon), this point lies on the back of the wrist, about three finger widths from the wrist crease, as shown. Giving pressure over this point has also been found to be extremely beneficial in overcoming heel pain. Further to this, I gave pressure over St-36, which lies four finger widths below the knee cap, one thumb width on the outside of the shin bone. This point strengthens the entire body, tones the muscles particularly when given in combination with Sp-6 (Three Yin Meeting Point) which is located above the ankle bone towards the inside of the leg on the back side about four finger widths above the ankle bone. This point is considered as the most potent point since it strengthens the yin of three meridians simultaneously. It is also considered to be best pressure point to overcome any gynecological problem, if any. Pregnant women should not press this point. I also pressed Sp-9, which lies on the inside of the leg, under the shin bone and is known to overcome any sort of edema in the lower part of the body.

Patients suffering from any sort of discomfort in the lumbosacral region respond tremendously to the points which fall on bladder meridian (B-23); B-40 (Command point) on the back of the knee; B-57; B-60; Gv-4 and Li-4, this trigger point (known as Adjoining Valley) over the large intestine meridian gives relief to pain in any part of the body by helping in circulating the Ch'i in the entire body. The precise location of these points has been shown in the figure.

Much to my surprise, the patient responded beyond my expectations. She was given treatment at around 10.30 am and at around 8.30 pm, she telephoned me to inform that she was feeling much better and that she had taken a pain-killer the previous day evening and thereafter she had not taken any pain-killer. Next day when she came for her session, she brought along with her, her mother too with certain problems. Her treatment lasted for around 14 or 15 sessions and she reported that she has taken only two pain-killers since she started treatment and that too within first four or five sessions. No pain-killer for the past 10 days. She further informed that she had stopped wearing the specially designed slipper, which she had been using for the last seven years to overcome the discomfort in her heel. As for her pain in the lumbosacral area, she retorted that doctor. I will have to try to locate the area that used to hurt me. At this stage, I advised her to stop the treatment and handed over a chart to her, with the intended pressure points to be pressed, in case the pain recurs. Also advised her to avoid lifting weight, forward-bending as also jumping from height, etc. This was done as during her treatment, it was felt that over her vertebral column, due to her improper posture, perhaps in her effort to ward off pain in that area, a buldge was felt around L4-L5 and S-1 area, an indicator of probable prolapsed disc problem at a later date.

□

Dietary and Yogic Tips for Musculoskeletal Disorders:

Lumbar Spondylosis; Cervical Spondylosis; Frozen Shoulder; Polyarthritis; Osteoarthritis; Rheumatoid arthritis; Lumbago, etc.

A. Diet Regime:

6.00 am — 100 gm Saunff; 100 gm Methi; 50 gm Alesi seeds (flex seeds); 20 gm Ajwain + 20 gm Ama Haldi Powder, 1 tsp powder with warm water.

6.30 am — 2-4 Munnakka; 8 Kishmish; 2-4 Badam; 2 Akhrot (soaked overnight).

9.00 am — Veg., Oats Daliya + 1 glass Ama Haldi (1/4 tsp) Milk.

11.00 am — Sprouts (Moong; Channa; Alfa-alfa; Methi; Mooth; tsp each+ lemon honey juice (1/4 tsp lemon+ 1 glass warm water)

12-1.00 pm — Boiled veg sabji + 1 multigrain wheat roti+ ½ cup Moong/Lal Masoor Dal) + fresh curds+salads)

5.00 pm — Carrot juice/Ashguard juice

8.00 pm — Veg soup + boiled vegetables + 200 gm papaya.

9.00 pm — Warm triphala ras) (1-1/2 tsp) with warm water.

B. Yoga Regime for Musculoskeletal Disorders:

1. Kapal Bati Kriya – 300 counts.
2. Asanas – Standing series:
   1. Katichakrasana with breath –

2. Tadasana while breathing
3. Trikonasana – breathing
4. Padhastasana (10 counts) followed by
5. Ardha Chakrasana (2 counts)
6. Ardha Katichakrasana (both sides)—breathing
7. Rekha Gati

Supine Series:

1. Uttanpadasana (30, 45)
2. Markatasana (Lumbar Stretch)
3. Setubandhasana

Prone Series:

1. Bhujangasana (Ardha/Pooran/Tiryank)
2. Shalabhasana
3. Naukasana

Sitting Series:

1. Vakrasana
2. Gomukhasana
3. Merudandasana
4. Ustrasana

Pranayaam:

1. Suryabhedan Pranayaam — (10 mins)
2. Anulom Vilom — (5 mins)
3. Bhramari — (24 rounds)
4. Aum — (24 rounds)
5. Maunn — (1 min)

□

Good Health and Immunity

When your dinner is simply soup:

A primary indication of health is how well your immune system defenses to fight off enemies, e.g. viruses and tumor cells.

Soup at dinner time is extremely healthy. Light meal at night reduces the digestive load on your body, leaving it free to regenerate, rejuvenate and heal while you sleep.

Foods that stimulate health:

Garlic; Mushrooms; Beta Carotene (Carrot, Spinach, Beetroot, Pumpkin, Sweet potato).

Vitamin C (Peppers, Broccoli), Cabbage, Spinach, Tomatoes;

Vitamin- E (Nuts, Oils), Zinc (Shell fish, Grains).

□

Some health conditions-Managed by Light Dinner

SOME HEALTH CONDITIONS THAT CAN BE MANAGED WHEN YOU LIGHTEN THE LAST MEAL OF THE DAY i.e. (Dinner)

1. Bronchial Asthma:

Hot, spicy, pungent foods can help clear the lungs and breathing passages. They do so by thinning mucus and encouraging it to move along. When we eat a hot food, our eyes tear up, nose begins to run. The same thing happens in our lungs, hot foods trigger nerve endings in the esophagus and stomach, causing the watery reactions.

A soup made with ginger, chili, pepper, raddish, black pepper, mustard and garlic have mucus-clearing activity, reducing airway inflammation and swelling. The hydration provided by the soup helps the body improve circulation and prevents the build-up of phlegm. Soups that contain onions and spinach have a therapeutic impact on the regeneration of cells and mucus membranes in reducing congestion.

2. Heart Patients–Cardiac Ailments:

To prevent attacks in the early morning hours, soup at dinner time should include garlic, turmeric, some oats (their soluble fiber helps lower cholesterol), low salt and vegetables like broccoli (its calcium content has a protective effect on the cardiac muscles). Barley, carrot, oats, soyabeans, onion, garlic, ginger are natural anti-oxidants, blood thinner and diuretic in nature which acts as cardiac tonic-lowering LDL (bad cholesterol) and raise HDL (good cholesterol).

3. Diabetes Mellitus:

Soup at dinner time along with boiled or steamed vegetables and papaya help in sugar control. Corriandar, garlic, onion, barley, beans, cabbage, broccoli (high chromium foods), mushrooms are beneficial in management of diabetes. Since what you eat has a major impact on blood sugar & insulin (the harmone that stimulates cells to absorb and store glucose (sugar), food is prime player in triggering, exacerbating and controlling diabetes. Thus broccoli, barley, mushrooms, whole grain contains high chromium (trace mineral) that seems to work wonder on blood sugar) by regulating blood sugar.

4. Obesity:

Food consumed at dinner just sits in the stomach, adding to weight gain because metabolism at night is sluggish. So eat your heavy meals at lunch time and stick to lentil soups with vegetables at dinner. Black channa and bean soup are good choice. Broccoli, cabbage, pumpkin, green, leafy vegetables, oats, barley are low calorific, improve metabolism, support immunity & assures guaranteed good health and weight loss.

5. Peptic Ulcers and Gastritis:

Stomach can be irritated by the foods that increase stomach acids. A diet plan that limits or does not include the food that irritates your stomach helps in management of ulcers, gastritis, one has to limit or avoid drinks and foods that cause symptoms, such as stomach pain, heartburn or indigestion.

Cabbage is an anti biotic. Cabbage contains gefarnate and carbenoxolone - compound used as anti-ulcer drug.

Herbal/Green tea is good, rich in anti-bacterial, anti-oxidant polyphenols called catechins.

Use of low fat cheese, yoghurt, tofu or soya products introducing proteins in diet.

Fruits and vegetables – carrot, broccoli, red/green peppers, beans, grapes, cabbage, apricots, kiwi fruit for their beta carotene and Vitamin C content, in order to protect the lining of the stomach and intestines.

Sunflower seeds/almonds are helpful due to their anti-oxidant and anti-inflammatory properties.

Curd/sprouts/soups in diet.

Foods to be avoided:

1. Milk }
2. Beer/alcohol } Interfere with your stomach
3. Smoking } lining and increase production
4. Coffee } of stomach acid.
5. Coca cola }
6. Red meat }

Eat Bananas and Plantains:

Bananas stimulate proliferation of cells and mucus that forms a strong barrier between the stomach lining and corrosive acids & prevents stomach damage. Plantain must be cooked before eating because they are too hard and tough to eat raw. Green plantains are considered more potent medicine for healing ulcers than ripe ones.

Consumption of Cabbage Juice:

Strengthens the stomach linings, resistance to acid attacks increases mucus activity, rejuvenating ulcerated cells, leading to healing fatty foods and dairy products:

They are harder to digest, so your body produces more stomach acid and aggravates condition, as such foods contains caffeine.

Note: Eating large meals requires the stomach to produce large amount of stomach acid. So, it is best to eat small meals. Ideally, have five to six meals a day, instead of two or three large ones.

□

Yog for Healthy Living

A. Kriya

1. Agnisar (5 min) empty stomach

Indications (Person can do)	Contra Indiacation (Person should Avoid)
1. Digestive problems	1. Cardiac (Heart) Patients
– Constipation	
– Indigestion	
2. Obesity	2. Hyper Tension (high B.P.)
3. Diabetes Mellitow	3. Hyperacidity
4. Abdominal Fat	4. Piles
	5. Kidney Patients

B. Asanas with Breathing – Start with three rounds of AUM Chanting

2. Kapal bathi (five min)

Supine Position

1. Hand in and out-breathing (five rounds)
2. Hand stretch breathing (five rounds)
3. Katichakrasana breathing (five rounds each)
4. Toe stand (Tadasana) breathing (five rounds)
5. Side ward stretch right and left (five rounds each)
6. Ardha chakrasana breathing (five rounds) (Backward bending)
7. Ardha kati Chakrasana breathing (three rounds each)

8. Trikonasana breathing (three rounds each)

Supine Position

1. *Shavasana (QRT):* Quick relaxation technique. (3 min) (Concentrate on up and down movement of abdomen and synchronize with breathing)

2. *AUM+OM charting*

- A – Chanting three rounds (by keeping bothhands over lower abdomen)
- U – Chanting three rounds (by keeping right hand over left-chest)
- M–chanting three rounds (by keeping both hands in stretched position over nape of neck)
- Finally, OM chanting – 9 rounds

3. *Setubandhasana breathing (three rounds)*

Prone position

1. Bhujangasana breathing (five rounds)
2. Makarasana/Balasana.

Sitting position

1. Paschimotanasana breathing (three rounds)
2. Pelvic stretch with breathing (three rounds)

C. PRANAYAMA

1

Bastrika
- Vyam (left nostril) (three min)
- Dakshin (right nostril) (three min)
- Madhyam (both nostril) (four min)
- (Quick fast/Inhalation and Exhalation)

2

Suryabedhan: (Inhalation through Right-nostril Exhalation through left nostril) 10 min

Indications: Obesity/Hypothyrodism/Diabetes/ Ashthma/Ortho problems/Neurological problems

Contra Indications: (Cardiac patient/Hyperacidity/ kidney problem/under weight (Hyperthyrodism)

3

Chandrabedan: (Inhalation through left nostril and Exhalation through right)

Good for High B.P./Heart patient/depression/ Hyperacidity

4. Anulom-vilom: (Alternate nostril breathing)

5 Bhramari : (5 min) Good for

1. Stress Relief
2. Anxiety
3. Voice Culture
4. Concentration
5. Confidence
6. Psychiatric problems

End the session by charting OM for three rounds

□

Dietary Management for Healthy Living

6 am : Water drinking (2-4 glasses) add ¼ tsp methi seeds, 1 Moonaka, 4-5 krishmish, 2 Badam, 1 Anjeer, 1 Akhroat Soaked overnight)

6.30 am : ½ Lemon, 1tsp honey, 1 glass water (Lemon honey juice)

7.30-8.30 am : 1 Glass butermilk + 15 min later any fruit preferably (Papaya/water-melon/Muskmelon/Apple/... etc.)

12 pm-1.30 pm : Salad+Boiled/Steamed vegetable Sabji 300-400 gms + 1–2 chokar pori+curd or Butter milk

4-5 pm : ½ Loki+ 1 cucumber+¼tsp lemonjuice, 1 Glass juice add 50 ml water

7.30-8.30 pm : Vegetable Soup+Vegetable Moong daliya+ Steamed Sabji+Papaya

9.30 pm : Warm milk

10 pm : Triphala water (10 days later on weekly once) (1 tsp) in luke warm water

Dietary tips for hypertension and cardiovascular disorders

1. Barley water 150 ml daily
2. Bottlegaurd and cucumber juice 150ml daily
3. Black grape juice 150 ml daily
4. Garlic (2-3 pods) daily

Rx. treatment

1. Hot foot bath (10-15 min) daily keep cold towel over head.

2. Multani mud application over abdomen 20 min daily
3. Multani mud bath once a week.

Dietary tips for Diabetes Mellitus

1. Barley water 150 ml daily
2. Bottle gaurd + Cucumber + Kerela juice 150 ml daily
3. Steamed Bitter gaurd (Kerela) pieces (2-4 pcs) daily
4. ½ tsp methi seeds daily
5. Vegetable soup with ¼ tsp Bhuni methi powder daily.
6. Papaya with one-fourth of outer peel
7. Jamun or Jamun seed powder 1tsp
8. Musumbi or Orange.

Rx. treatment

1. Gastro-Hepatic pack (20-30 min daily)
2. Hot foot bath (10-15 min) Simultaneously Ice massage over liver area (10 min)

Dietary Management/Tips for Renal Problems (Kidney problems)

1. Barley water 150 ml daily.
2. Bottlegourd juice 150 ml daily.
3. Raddish juice ½ cup daily add 50 ml water to juice.
4. Avoid Dal/Proteins introduce steamed vegetables.

(Rx) treatment

1. Hot foot bath (10-15 min) daily once.
2. Kidney pack (20-30 min).

Dietary Management /Tips for the eye Disorders/Health of Eyes

1. Carrot juice 150 ml daily
2. Black grape juice 150 ml daily
3. Salads (raw salads)
4. Raw diet (sprouts-mung/channa/Alfa-Alfa)
5. Raw Vegetables. (cucumber/beetroot/carrot/raddish)

6. ¼ tsp methi seeds, 2 moonaka, 4-5 kishmish, 1 Anjeer, 2 Badam, 1 Akroat Soaked over night daily.

(Rx)

1. Eye wash (using normal/lukewarm water or Triphala water)
2. Eye Exercises daily once for 20-30 mins.
3. Deep breathing/pranayama daily.
4. Cold ice pack over eye circles/cucumber pack.

□□□

Reflex Centres on the feet

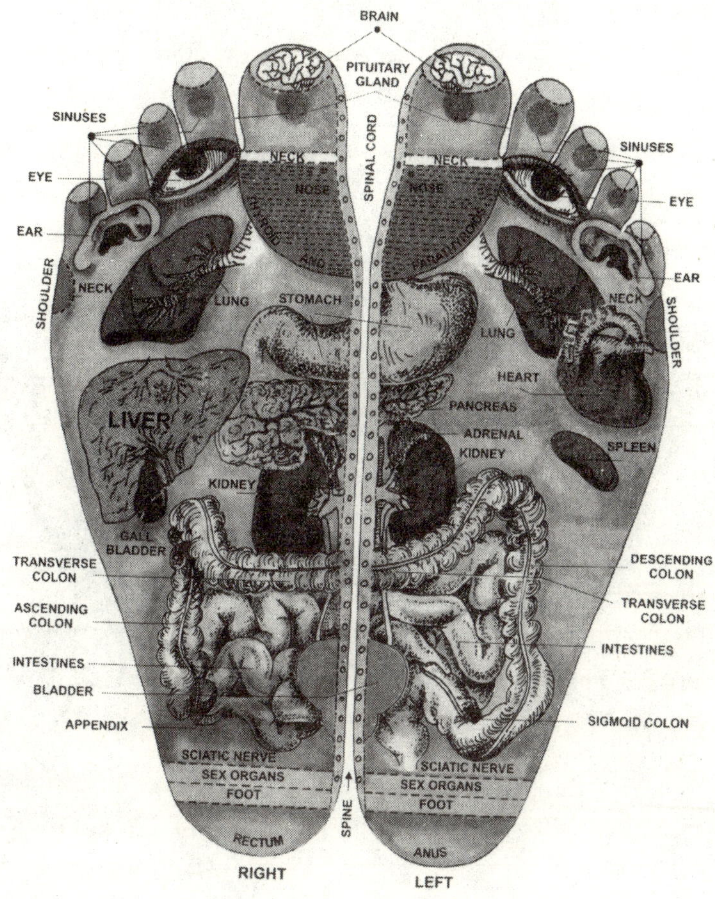

Adopted with thanks from the book
Acupressure Do-it-yourself therapy by my Guruji
Dr. Attar Singh

Reflex Centres on the Hands

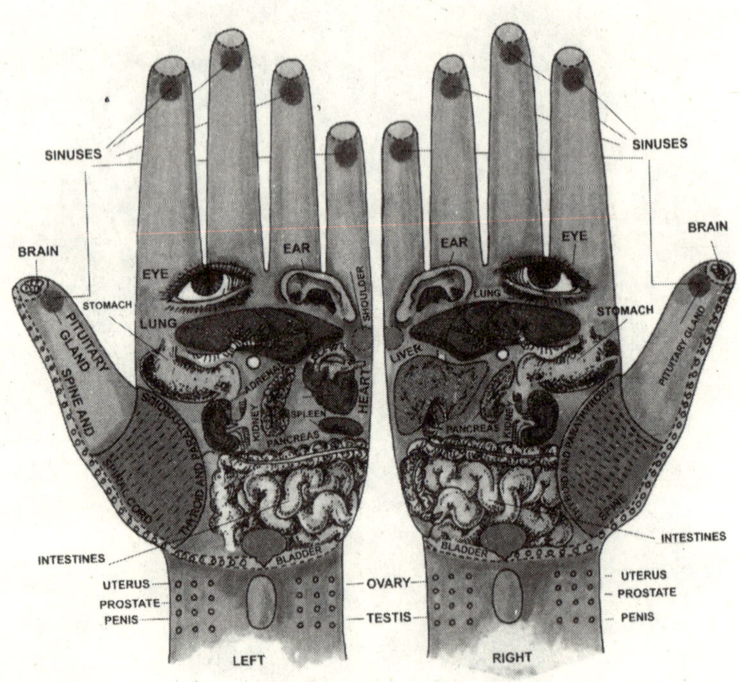

Adopted with thanks from the book
Acupressure Do-it-yourself therapy by my Guruji
Dr. Attar Singh